OSTEOPOROSIS

The book I wish I'd had when I was diagnosed

LISA POCIUS MD

Medical Disclaimer: This book is provided for educational and informational purposes only and is not intended as medical advice, diagnosis, or treatment. The content is not a substitute for professional medical judgment or consultation with a qualified healthcare professional. Readers should consult their own physician or other licensed healthcare provider regarding any medical condition, treatment, medication, or health-related decision.

Trademark Acknowledgment: FRAX® and FRAXplus® are trademarks of © Osteoporosis Research Limited, Reprinted with permission from ORL. All rights reserved.

Drug/Product Mention Disclaimer: Reference to specific medications in this book is for educational, informational, and illustrative purposes only and does not constitute endorsement, recommendation, or preference by the author or publisher.

Published by Lisa Pocius, MD
www.mybone.health

ISBN: 979-8-9955646-0-7 (paperback)
ISBN: 979-8-9955646-2-1 (large-print hardcover)
ISBN: 979-8-9955646-1-4 (eBook)

Text: Lisa Pocius, MD
Illustrations: Tuba Shahbaz
Cover and interior formatting by KUHN Design Group | kuhndesigngroup.com
Editing: Claire Dunn

To my mother,
who is stronger than she knows.

ACKNOWLEDGMENTS

This book benefited from feedback from a team of early readers, work with Claude (yes, that Claude), and polish by my editor, Claire Dunn.

I'm grateful for my medical team, Dr. Kalelkar, Dr. Katz Small, Dr. Said, and, especially, Dr. Brander. Their support through my own osteoporosis journey inspired me to write this book.

Most of all, I need to thank my husband, John, and our children, Sofia, Mia, and Johnny, for their support and patience. I really was writing a book all those nights on the laptop.

CONTENTS

WHO THIS BOOK IS FOR

If you've just learned that your bones aren't as strong as you thought, this book is for you. It doesn't matter whether you discovered your diagnosis through a routine screening or, like me, through unexpected fractures. It also doesn't matter whether your doctor used the word "osteoporosis" or "osteopenia" (mild bone loss). These aren't two separate diseases; they're points along a spectrum of bone density loss. The same strategies that help someone with severe osteoporosis also help someone with mild osteopenia prevent things from getting worse.

I wrote this book as both a physician and a patient. I know what it's like to sit in an exam room feeling frightened and overwhelmed, wondering what this diagnosis means for your future. I also know, from decades of medical practice, that knowledge is power. My goal is to give you both the reassurance that you can live well with this condition and the concrete, evidence-based guidance to actually do it.

HOW THIS BOOK IS ORGANIZED

Before you begin, I want to give you a quick map of where we're going together. This book is organized into three parts, and my personal story is woven throughout. You'll hear how I discovered my diagnosis, how I navigated the emotional fallout, and what I learned at every stage of my recovery. I share my experience not because my story is unique, but because I want you to know that the person writing these pages has walked this road and come out stronger on the other side.

Part 1: Discovery is where we start. After my diagnosis story in Chapter 1, I take you straight into the emotional journey in Chapter 2. The fear, grief, and anxiety that follow a bone loss diagnosis are real, and they deserve attention before we get into the science. From there, we build your foundation of knowledge: how your bones actually build, break down, and rebuild (Chapter 3); how to read your DEXA scan and understand your T-scores and FRAX® risk assessment (Chapter 4); what osteoporotic fractures look like and how they're treated (Chapter 5); and the hidden factors that may be quietly stealing your bone strength right now (Chapter 6).

Part 2: Treatment and Active Management is where knowledge turns into action. This is the heart of the book, covering the three pillars of fighting back against bone loss: exercise that actually builds bone (Chapter 7); nutrition strategies, including the best sources of calcium and vitamin D (Chapter 8); and a thorough guide to medication options, so you can have informed conversations with your doctor (Chapter 9). We close this section with practical advice on working with your healthcare team and advocating for yourself (Chapter 10).

Part 3: Living Well with Osteoporosis brings it all together with strategies for living safely and fully, from fall prevention to staying active without fear (Chapter 11). Finally, Chapter 12 (30-Day Action Plan) gives you a concrete week-by-week roadmap if you've just been diagnosed.

Finally, the resources at the end of this book are designed to be just as useful as the chapters themselves. You'll find **Final Thoughts**, with reflections on what it truly means to be strong; a **Frequently Asked Questions** section covering the most common questions about everything from calcium supplements to medication side effects; a **Glossary**, with pronunciation guides and definitions for the medical terminology you'll encounter; and **endnotes throughout**, so you can explore the research behind every recommendation.

You don't have to read this book cover to cover. If you've just been diagnosed and need to act now, start with the 30-Day Action Plan and then come back to fill in the details, or pick the chapters on the topics you have the most questions about. If you're an information-first person like me, start at Chapter 1 and let the story unfold. Either way, everything you need is here.

PART 1

DISCOVERY

CHAPTER 1

MY UNEXPECTED DIAGNOSIS

A Physician's Osteoporosis Story

My journey with osteoporosis, or at least of experiencing its devastating effects, began thanks to my standard-size goldendoodle, Finnegan. He's a big dog. He's a sweet dog. He's a dog that doesn't have much impulse control. One unexpectedly warm early October day, I took him out with me to dig up a few weeds near the street. It was beautiful outside, and I took my time figuring out which plants to pull and which to leave in a few more weeks for the last few bees buzzing around the yard.

That's when Finnegan saw a man walking a dog down the road toward us. I hadn't seen the man, and Finnegan's jerk on the leash was totally unexpected. He yanked me right up off my feet, and I landed square on both elbows. He then pulled me clear across the parkway toward the other dog, and finally, I had to let go lest I get dragged across the pavement and into the road. If it had been a cartoon, it might have been comical, and my elbows would have cut railroad tracks into the grass. Finnegan, now loose and barking, ran in circles around the man and his dog.

Embarrassed and worried about the man feeling unsafe (despite my goofy dog being harmless), I got up, brushed myself off, collected Finnegan, and apologized profusely. The man was more worried about me after such a fall. I assured him I was okay. After all, I was only 55; I wasn't an old woman. I wasn't frail. I felt an odd pinch in my upper back, and my knees and elbows were scraped, but no harm done. After cleaning myself up, I took some ibuprofen and went on with my day.

Little did I know, but this seemingly minor incident would be the catalyst that revealed a condition that had been silently developing in my bones for years. The fall didn't cause my osteoporosis; it simply exposed the weakness that was already there.

WARNING SIGNS

With a busy job as a medical director and a family of teenagers who needed me, I forgot about the fall. Then, in November, I started noticing a worsening ache in my back, right between my shoulder blades. It didn't seem too unusual, as I've always had stiff muscles in my upper back and carried tension in my neck and shoulders. When my daughter suggested a massage, I said, "That's a great idea." I usually like deep tissue massages, but this time, when the massage therapist got to the middle of my back, I felt a sudden pain. Typically, when a massage therapist puts deep pressure on my paraspinal muscles (those long muscles that go up and down alongside the spine), it feels great. This time, it hurt a lot! Hindsight is 20/20, of course, and I realize now I should have told him to stop. Instead, I let him keep going, thinking it was only painful because he was working some knots out of my muscles.

The pain went on through the holiday season. I still managed to get through the buzz of holiday parties, but the deep ache just would not go away. It got worse each day. In January, I thought perhaps one of my ribs was subluxed (out of place) and causing pain to radiate to my back. I had the excellent physical therapist in our clinic do some therapy to realign it. The experience was more painful than times he'd worked on me previously, which should have been a sign to me that something was wrong.

As I was slowly getting up off the table, the therapist remarked that he didn't want to try to adjust me anymore; the tenderness I was experiencing seemed to be coming from my spine, not a rotated rib or spasming muscle. "Have you ever had a DEXA scan?" he asked (a dual-energy X-ray absorptiometry or DEXA scan is an imaging test that measures bone mineral density). "No," I laughed, brushing off his comment. Being a doctor, I knew that it wasn't an unreasonable question to ask a woman in her 50s with back pain, but the possibility of osteoporosis seemed, well, ridiculous. I was much too young and active to worry about that. I did agree to get a quick X-ray; everything in my back looked fine, except for a little kyphosis, or forward curve of the spine, in my mid-back. I chalked that up to poor posture.

Did You Know? Only about one-third of vertebral fractures ever come to medical attention. Most happen silently, with no obvious symptoms, and go undiagnosed for years.[1]

SEEKING ANSWERS

Finally, the pain became so unbearable that I stopped doctoring myself and got myself in to see my own doctor. She agreed that the pain I had was severe and unusual. An MRI (magnetic resonance imaging) was the next step; when performed on the back, this test can visualize the soft tissues, including muscles and vertebral disks; it also can show damage on the inside of the bones of the spine. When the MRI of my spine was finished, the technician, who'd been rather unconcerned when asking me to "hop" onto the table, ran over to help me off the table as if I were 100 years old. Hmm, I didn't like that! The next day, the results popped up on my phone: I had not one but four compression fractures in my thoracic vertebrae. T6, T7, T8, and T9, which are in the upper to middle back, showed crush-type changes and a lot of edema (swelling and fluid buildup) inside the bones. No wonder I was in so much pain. Luckily, there were no bone fragments putting pressure on my spinal cord.

FACING THE FEAR

The momentary relief of at least knowing why I was in pain was quickly overshadowed by the fear of what could have caused those fractures. As a doctor, I knew very well that fractures like this after just a minimal-impact injury could well be from cancer or another type of bone disease. In fact, I knew that if I'd been in my 40s, those would have been the more likely reasons for fractures like this. I was in my 50s, though, and about seven years postmenopausal, so osteoporosis was the probable cause. I just couldn't wrap

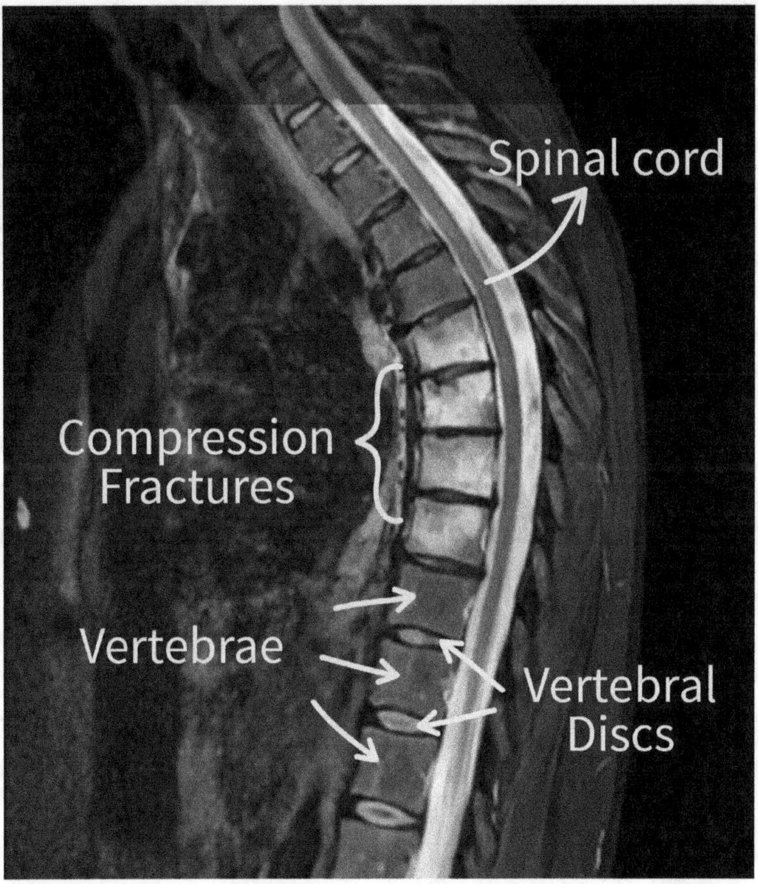

Figure 1.1: MRI of my thoracic spine (February 2025). The bracket highlights compression fractures at T6–T9 with bone marrow edema (the bright signal indicates acute injury). These fractures weren't visible on plain X-ray.

my head around the fact that I might be experiencing something that I didn't think would happen for another few decades. My fears of cancer kept me up at night and scared my family.

In the following three months, while tests came back negative for cancer and other bone diseases, I suffered blinding pain that made me sweaty and nauseous. I started thinking about patients I'd cared for with painful vertebral fractures. Had I been empathetic enough? Not everyone experiences pain with vertebral fractures, but when they do, it can be debilitating. There's nothing like experiencing a condition yourself to understand it.

Thankfully, I was able to take some time away from work. I'm fortunate to have paid sick leave and an understanding boss. For a while, I couldn't even telework; I couldn't sit up long enough.

THE LONG ROAD TO RECOVERY

By the time we realized I had the fractures, it was considered too late to have the most common aggressive treatment for compression fractures: kyphoplasty. During this procedure, a body-safe cement is injected into the vertebrae; it kills the pain and often even "puffs" the vertebrae back up. At first, I was limited to being up off the bed or couch for only a few hours a day, and I was unable to lift anything heavier than a cup of coffee or bend down to pick something off the floor. When I was up and around, I wore a hard back brace that reminded me a little of an exoskeleton.

It was a long, slow healing process. Eventually, after several months, I turned the corner and the pain slowly lessened. Of course, I'd come through injuries and illness before, but this time, I knew I'd have to make some substantial changes to heal fully. I changed my diet, began weight-bearing exercise, and started strong bone-building medication.

A NEW REALITY

Those osteoporotic fractures, though, came with a lot of baggage that I didn't expect. Something about feeling like I was weak in my bones, in my very core, was unsettling. Suddenly, I felt weak and fragile. I was afraid of falling. I started rethinking my activities. There really was a sense of loss: an invisible one, but a real one.

TURNING LOSS INTO ACTION

For me, the best way to deal with a sense of loss is to meet it head-on with action. Doing the research and authoring this book has helped me tremendously. My hope, whether you've been surprised by fractures, just learned you have osteoporosis from a screening test, or received a diagnosis of osteopenia and want to prevent things from getting worse, is that this book will help you, too. Remember, osteopenia and osteoporosis aren't two separate diseases; they're points along a spectrum of bone density loss, and the strategies for protecting your bones apply across that entire range.

KEY TAKEAWAYS

- Osteoporosis is a silent disease that often reveals itself only through a fracture from low-impact trauma.
- Estimates suggest that one in two to one in three women over 50 will experience an osteoporotic fracture, which are sometimes silent and sometimes very painful.[2,3]
- Taking informed action after diagnosis is the most powerful response to this condition.

CHAPTER 2

THE EMOTIONAL JOURNEY

From Shock to Strength

In the weeks and months following my diagnosis, I expected the hardest part would be the physical recovery. I was wrong. While I lay on the couch in my back brace, unable to sit up for more than a few hours, the emotional weight of what had happened began to settle in. The emotional journey, encompassing fear, vulnerability, and the gradual rebuilding of confidence, proved just as challenging and just as important as any medical intervention.

My osteoporosis diagnosis caught me completely off guard, and the shock was immediate and overwhelming. Even as a physician who should have known better, I simply didn't have bone health on my radar. I was 55, active, and busy, not someone I pictured as being "fragile." That label felt foreign and frightening. Whether your DEXA report says "osteoporosis" or "osteopenia," the emotional weight of learning your bones are weaker than you thought hits just as hard. In some ways, osteopenia can feel even more confusing, because you're left wondering whether you should be worried or relieved.

Shock quickly gave way to fear. As I shared in the previous chapter, I was terrified that the compression fractures were from undiagnosed cancer or some rare disease I'd never considered. The weeks of waiting for test results felt endless, filled with anxious internet searches and worst-case scenario planning. Even my medical knowledge couldn't shield me from a very human response to uncertainty about my health.

COMMON EMOTIONAL RESPONSES

As I talked with other people who'd been through similar diagnoses, I learned that my experience wasn't unique at all. Research shows that people diagnosed with osteoporosis frequently go through predictable psychological responses that can significantly impact their quality of life and treatment success.

Anxiety is perhaps the most common reaction, and I felt it acutely. The fear of falling became constant background noise: "Will I fracture if I trip?" "Can I still travel safely?" "Should I avoid stairs altogether while I'm healing?" This anxiety often leads to activity restriction, which ironically weakens bones further, which in turn increases fall risk, creating a vicious cycle. I even found myself anxious about whether people could see the new little forward curve in my upper back.

Depression can follow, especially after fractures. The combination of chronic pain, loss of independence, and changed body image creates overwhelming challenges. I watched some people withdraw from activities they once enjoyed, compounding both their physical and their emotional problems.

Loss of self-esteem may strike particularly hard. For those of us who've always prided ourselves on being strong and independent, osteoporosis can feel like a fundamental betrayal by our own bodies. The invisible nature of bone loss makes this especially challenging; I looked the same from the outside but felt fundamentally different inside.

Social isolation often develops as people limit their activities or withdraw from social roles. Unlike visible conditions, which others can readily understand and accommodate, osteoporosis requires people to explain invisible limitations and fears that may seem disproportionate to friends and family.

CHANGING HOW YOU THINK ABOUT YOURSELF

For me, perhaps the most challenging aspect involved the transition from seeing myself as a "healthy person" to accepting life as "someone with a chronic condition." This identity shift felt abrupt and disorienting, especially since my diagnosis followed an unexpected fracture rather than a gradual recognition of symptoms.

I found myself moving differently and thinking differently about my body's capabilities. Simple activities, like reaching for items on high shelves or bending to pick up dropped objects, required conscious thought and planning. I was hyperaware of my back in ways I'd never experienced before.

The psychological impact proved as limiting as any physical restriction. Some days, I caught myself avoiding activities not because they were dangerous but because the fear of potential consequences felt overwhelming.

A NOTE FOR MEN WITH OSTEOPOROSIS

The psychological burden of this diagnosis can be particularly challenging for men. Many men describe feeling embarrassed or emasculated by having what's widely perceived as a "women's disease." This stigma can prevent men from discussing their diagnosis with friends or family, creating additional isolation. Some men report that their healthcare providers dismissed their concerns or seemed surprised by the diagnosis. If you're a man reading this, know that osteoporosis is not a reflection of your masculinity; it's a medical condition affecting an estimated one to two million American men, and likely many more who remain undiagnosed.[4,5] The courage to address it head-on is strength, not weakness.

> **Did You Know?** While 90% of physicians would screen a 65-year-old woman for osteoporosis, only 22% would screen a 74-year-old man. Yet men are twice as likely as women to die within a year of a hip fracture. This screening gap costs lives.[6,7]

WORKING THROUGH THE GRIEF PROCESS

Looking back, I recognize that I went through something resembling grief; I was mourning the loss of my previous sense of invulnerability and the carefree relationship I'd had with my body.

There was denial: "This can't be right; the test must be wrong." Anger followed: "Why me? I've tried to take care of myself." Bargaining came next: "If I do everything perfectly now, maybe I can completely reverse this." Then depression crept in: "My body is failing me, and there's nothing I can do about it."

Eventually, acceptance emerged. It initially manifested as resignation, but it soon became the foundation for empowerment. Once I stopped fighting the diagnosis and started working with it constructively, I could channel my energy into positive action rather than futile resistance. That acceptance marked a real turning point in my emotional journey.

FINDING MY PATH FORWARD

The emotional journey with osteoporosis isn't just about coping with a medical diagnosis; it's about rebuilding confidence and reclaiming your sense of personal agency. Through my own experience and conversations with others, several strategies proved particularly helpful.

Education functioned as emotional medicine. The more I understood bone biology and treatment options, the less frightening the condition became. Knowledge replaced vague fears with concrete, actionable plans. Understanding that osteoporosis is manageable and that effective treatments exist helped shift my mindset from victim to active participant.

Connection with others proved invaluable. Whether through informal conversations with friends who'd faced similar challenges or via online communities of people managing osteoporosis, sharing the experience reduced my isolation significantly. I was surprised to discover how many people in my circle had dealt with similar diagnoses or concerns about bone health.

Focusing on controllable factors became liberating. While I couldn't change my age, genetics, or past bone loss, I could absolutely control my nutrition, exercise consistency, medication adherence, and safety measures. This shift, from feeling victimized by circumstances to actively managing my health, proved to be transformative.

REFRAMING THE NARRATIVE

Instead of viewing osteoporosis as evidence of weakness or failure, I began seeing my diagnosis and treatment as proof of my commitment to future health. Every calcium supplement, every balance exercise, and even every dose of medication became an act of self-care and determination rather than a reminder of limitation.

I started celebrating small victories. The first wall push-up without back pain felt monumental. The first long walk without needing a pain pill represented genuine progress. These weren't dramatic fitness achievements, but they were meaningful steps toward rebuilding my bone bank and my confidence.

DISCOVERING UNEXPECTED BENEFITS

Living with osteoporosis has brought insights and even gifts I never anticipated. I pay attention to my body now in ways I never did before. I'm more intentional about movement and more mindful about nutrition. I'm more grateful for my current mobility and independence.

The diagnosis forced me to confront my own mortality, but in doing so, it also clarified my priorities. I stopped making excuses about exercise: no more "I'm too busy" or "I'll start tomorrow." My bones needed me to move, so I moved. This clarity of purpose improved other areas of my health as well.

I became an unexpected advocate for bone health among my friends and patients. People now ask me about calcium supplements and exercise routines. I encourage acquaintances to get DEXA scans and discuss osteoporosis prevention with their doctors. In helping others understand and prevent osteoporosis, I've found purpose and meaning in my diagnosis.

WHEN PROFESSIONAL SUPPORT HELPS

The emotional impact of osteoporosis can be significant enough to warrant professional attention. Counseling and support groups can dramatically improve quality of life by helping to reduce anxiety and depression, and by providing practical strategies for managing fear and activity restriction.

Stress management techniques benefit both mental health and bone health, since chronic stress elevates cortisol levels, which can accelerate bone loss. Practices like meditation and deep breathing exercises improved my emotional well-being while potentially supporting my skeletal health.

Professional guidance also helped me address psychological barriers to exercise, like fear of hurting myself by falling or doing an exercise incorrectly. Sometimes, having an objective perspective made all the difference in working through challenges.

MOVING FORWARD WITH HARD-WON WISDOM

About one year after my diagnosis, I can honestly say that while I wouldn't choose to have osteoporosis, it has changed me in several positive ways. I'm more attuned to my overall health, more intentional about self-care, and more appreciative of my body's capabilities and resilience.

The fear hasn't disappeared entirely; I still think twice before stepping on icy sidewalks or reaching for something on a high shelf. But that awareness has evolved into wisdom rather than paralyzing anxiety. I take reasonable precautions without letting fear dictate my life choices.

I've learned that strength isn't just about bone density or muscle mass. True strength also encompasses adaptability and the courage to face health challenges directly and constructively. My bones may be more fragile than they once were, but my spirit has grown stronger through this experience.

HOPE AND ENCOURAGEMENT FOR OTHERS

If you're reading this in the early days of your own osteoporosis journey, know that the initial shock and fear will ease with time and knowledge. The overwhelming feeling of vulnerability will give way to a sense of empowerment as you take concrete action.

You are not broken. You are not weak. You are someone who now possesses valuable knowledge about your bone health that many people lack. You can take proactive steps to protect your future mobility and independence in ways that uninformed people cannot.

Your diagnosis may feel like an ending, but it can also mark the beginning of a more intentional and empowered approach to health and aging. The emotional journey takes time, patience with yourself, and sometimes professional support, but it can lead to a place of greater strength and wisdom than you might imagine possible right now.

Our bones may form the foundation of our physical structure, but resilience and determination form the foundation of how we respond to any challenge life presents. And those foundations, unlike our bone density, remain entirely within our control to strengthen and develop.

Processing the emotional aspects of my diagnosis proved essential for what came next. Once I'd worked through the initial shock and fear, I found myself hungry to understand what had actually happened inside my body. How had my bones failed me so completely without any warning? During those long recovery days, I dove back into the medical science I'd once studied, and what I discovered about the secret life of our skeletons changed everything I thought I knew.

KEY TAKEAWAYS

- Fear, anxiety, and loss of confidence are normal emotional responses to an osteoporosis or osteopenia diagnosis and can significantly impact quality of life.
- The fear of falling often leads to reduced activity, which ironically weakens bones further and increases fall risk, creating a harmful cycle.
- Developing psychological resilience through education, support systems, and gradually rebuilding confidence is as important as physical treatment.

CHAPTER 3

YOUR SKELETON'S SECRET LIFE

How Bones Build, Break Down, and Rebuild

During those long months of recovery, when I was wearing my back brace and moving like someone much older than my 55 years, I had plenty of time to think. As a physician, I'd learned about bones back in medical school, but honestly, I'd forgotten many of the details. What I did remember felt abstract: textbook knowledge disconnected from what was happening in my own body. So, I immersed myself in the research, rediscovering the science I'd once studied but never really understood on a personal level.

What I found renewed my appreciation for the complexity of our bones. If you've ever seen a skeleton in a museum or a doctor's office, it looks so static: clean white sticks frozen in time, like a Halloween decoration. But that couldn't be further from the truth. Our bones are alive. They're bustling with activity, constantly rebuilding themselves like a construction site that never shuts down.

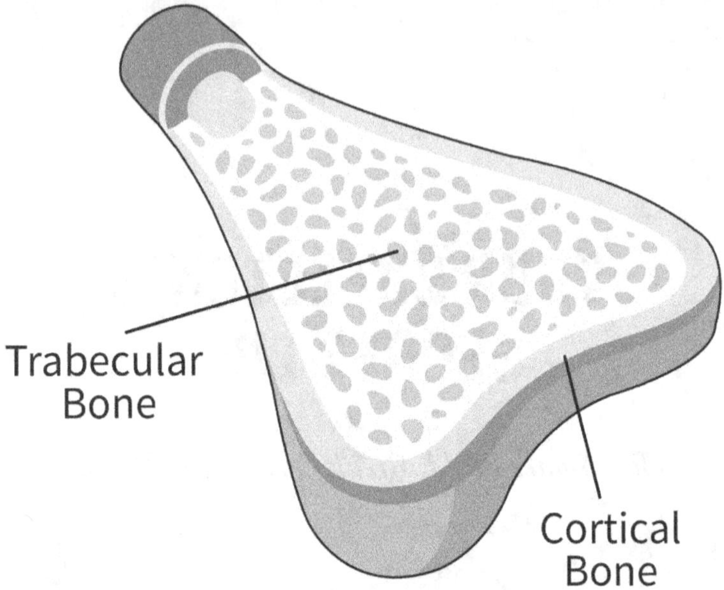

Figure 3.1: Cross-section of bone showing the dense outer cortical layer and the spongy inner trabecular (cancellous) bone.

I started thinking of my skeleton differently. My bones weren't just the scaffolding holding me up; they were living tissues with their own blood supply, sending chemical signals throughout my body. They housed the bone marrow that made every blood cell in my body. Pretty remarkable when you think about it.

THE BIOLOGY OF BONES

The skeleton has two main types of bone tissue, and understanding the difference helped me make sense of what had gone wrong in my own body. The outer shell is called cortical bone. Think of it like the walls of a house: dense and strong, making up about 80% of your skeleton's weight. This cortical bone is what gives you the structural strength to walk, run, and live your life without collapsing.

Inside, you have what's called spongy bone (doctors call it cancellous or trabecular bone), which creates a honeycomb-like network. This lighter, more delicate structure, full of developing blood cells, is especially abundant in your spine, hips, and ribs: all the bones that are most likely to fracture from osteoporosis. It's only 20% of your skeleton's weight, but it has a much larger surface area and is far more biologically active than the dense outer bone.

This design isn't accidental. If your entire skeleton were made of dense cortical bone, you'd be too heavy to move easily. Plus, you'd

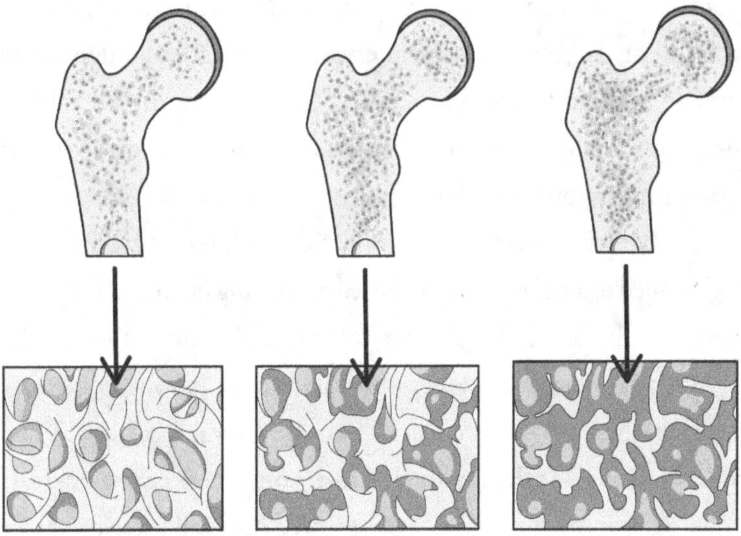

Figure 3.2: Comparison of the progression from normal bone density (left) to osteoporotic bone (right). Trabecular bone loses its dense honeycomb structure, leaving bones fragile and prone to fracture.

lose the marrow spaces where your blood cells form. That apparent "weakness" of spongy bone? It's actually evolutionary genius.

Learning this made me reconsider my spine fractures. Those four vertebrae collapsed from the inside out. The fractures started in the delicate honeycomb structure, which had quietly weakened while I went about my busy life, completely unaware.

UNDERSTANDING YOUR PERSONAL BONE BANK

The metaphor that helped me the most was thinking of bones as a bank, and specifically a calcium bank. This helped me understand what had been happening in my body for years before that fateful day with Finnegan.

Your skeleton stores 99% of your body's calcium. Maintaining the right calcium levels in your blood isn't optional; it's literally life or death. Your heart, nerves, and muscles all depend on precise calcium levels to function. So, when your blood calcium drops even slightly, your body doesn't hesitate to make a withdrawal from your bone bank.

The bank has two types of employees working around the clock. Cells called osteoblasts are like the tellers making deposits. They build new bone by first laying down a soft protein scaffold, then hardening it with calcium and other minerals to create strong bone tissue.

Then there are the osteoclasts, the withdrawal specialists. When your body needs calcium for vital functions, these cells quickly dissolve old bone tissue and release the stored minerals into your bloodstream. Osteoclasts are also the demolition crew that clears away old, worn-out bone to make room for fresh, strong replacements.

When I learned I had osteoporosis, I pictured my osteoclasts working overtime: too enthusiastic, like Finnegan yanking on that leash. Demolition without enough reconstruction.

This remodeling process never stops. Even in healthy adults, about 10% of your skeleton is remodeled each year, though the rate varies by bone type and location.[8],[9] It's like having contractors constantly renovating your house while you're still living in it, demolishing old sections and building new ones to keep everything structurally sound.

> **Did You Know?** Osteoclasts can break down bone in just four to six weeks, but osteoblasts need three to five months to rebuild it. In osteoporosis, this mismatch means bone is lost faster than it can be replaced.[10]

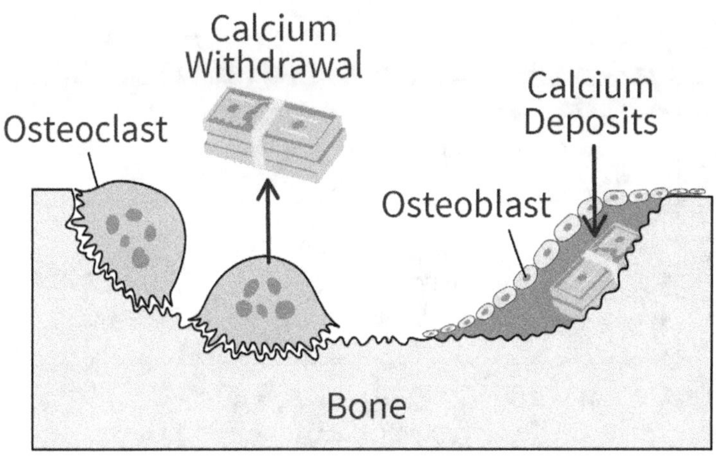

Figure 3.3: The "bone bank" metaphor. Osteoclasts make withdrawals by breaking down bone, while osteoblasts make deposits by building new bone matrix.

HOW YOUR ACCOUNT BALANCE CHANGES OVER TIME

Understanding how bone density changes throughout life helped me realize that my fractures weren't just bad luck; they were the result of decades of gradual changes I hadn't even noticed.

Think of childhood and adolescence as your peak years for bone density deposits. You accumulate about 90% of your peak bone mass by your late teens, with full peak density typically reached in your mid- to late 20s.[11],[12] This is when good nutrition and exercise can really pay dividends, building the strongest possible foundation for later life.

I thought about my own teenagers and realized I should be having conversations with them about their bone health. Because honestly, at their age, I hadn't been thinking about my bones at all. Who does?

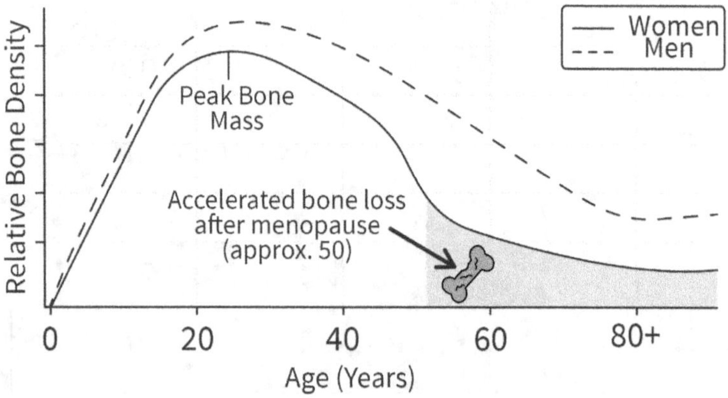

Figure 3.4: Bone density changes over the lifespan. Note the higher peak bone mass in men and the rapid decline in women following menopause.

Your 20s and early 30s are like the peak of your career: you reach your highest lifetime bone density, usually between ages 25 and 30. After that, you're essentially living off your savings, with small annual withdrawals that gradually accelerate over time.

BONE DENSITY CHANGES IN WOMEN VS. MEN

Women have some protection against bone loss through midlife. Estrogen acts like a good financial adviser, helping slow the withdrawals from your bone bank. But menopause? That's like losing your financial adviser overnight. The sudden drop in estrogen can trigger dramatic bone loss; in women who lose bone rapidly, that can mean as much as 20% over just 5–10 years. That's a lot! It's no wonder that so many women first discover osteoporosis in their 50s and 60s.[13]

Men typically have a different experience with bone loss. They generally build bigger, denser bones to start with, which provides a structural advantage; studies show that men have anywhere from 20 to 30% greater bone density than women, though differences vary by skeletal site and how those sites are measured. Testosterone provides bone protection in a similar way to estrogen's role in women, but the decline is more gradual compared with the sudden drop women experience at menopause. This means men typically develop osteoporosis about 10 years later than women. However, this later onset can be a double-edged sword: when men do develop osteoporosis, they often face delays in diagnosis because both they and their doctors assume it's a "women's disease." This delay means men often aren't diagnosed until after they've already experienced a fracture.[14]

WHEN WITHDRAWALS HAPPEN

This is key to understanding osteoporosis: your body always prioritizes short-term survival over long-term bone strength. If your blood calcium drops, your body will pull what it needs from your bones without asking permission. It doesn't care if this leaves your skeleton weakened; it cares about keeping your heart beating and your muscles functioning today.

This means that poor calcium intake, inadequate vitamin D (which helps you absorb calcium), or other factors that disrupt calcium balance can force your skeleton to become an unwilling donor. For years, my bones had been making these difficult choices, gradually becoming more fragile as they sacrificed their own integrity to keep the rest of my body functioning.

Understanding this helped me realize that my fall with Finnegan wasn't the cause of my problems; it was simply the final straw that revealed a weakness that had been building for years.

As I spent those quiet recovery days learning about my bones' secret life, I gained a new respect for the constant activity in my skeleton and was eager to know exactly how much strength I had left. That's when my doctor scheduled my first DEXA scan: my official bone bank statement.

KEY TAKEAWAYS

- Your bones are living tissue that constantly remodel themselves, with about 10% of your skeleton being completely renewed each year.
- Peak bone mass is typically reached in your 20s to 30s, after which gradual bone loss begins; this accelerates significantly after menopause for women while remaining gradual for men.
- Your body prioritizes short-term survival over long-term bone strength, pulling calcium from your bones whenever blood calcium levels drop.

CHAPTER 4

DECIPHERING YOUR DEXA SCAN

T-Scores, FRAX, and What Your Numbers Mean

Just as you can't manage your finances without knowing your account balance, you can't effectively manage bone health without understanding your bone density. Your DEXA scan is your official bone bank statement, showing you exactly where you stand and whether you've been losing bone strength over time.

I learned this the hard way. Like most people, I'd been walking around completely unaware of my bone health status. Osteoporosis earned its reputation as the "silent disease" because bone loss happens gradually, without symptoms, until that first fracture forces the discovery. It's like quietly draining your checking account until, one day, your debit card gets declined at the grocery store.

At least one-third of all women over 50 in the United States will experience an osteoporotic fracture. They're more common than breast cancer. But unlike cancer survivors, who often regain full health, only 40% of people with hip fractures (the most serious type of osteoporotic fracture) ever return to their previous level of independence. These fractures can profoundly impact quality of life through chronic pain, height loss, and fear of falling.[15,16] For something so common and devastating, it's shocking how little we talk about preventing it.

The statistics I discovered during my research were sobering. More than half of adults over 50 in the United States have osteopenia or osteoporosis; that's about 45 million Americans walking around with weakened bones. Most have no idea until a fracture announces the problem in the most painful way possible.[17,18]

EARLY WARNING SIGNS YOU MIGHT MISS

While DEXA scanning gives you the definitive measurement, sometimes, your body drops subtle hints about bone problems before you get tested. I wish I'd paid attention to some of these signs earlier.

Receding gums can signal jawbone loss. **Weakened grip strength**, surprisingly, predicts fracture risk quite well: a new and marked inability to open jars can signal possible bone density problems. **Brittle, easily broken nails** might suggest nutritional deficiencies that also affect bones.

Loss of height is a big red flag. If you've shrunk more than an inch and a half from your peak adult height, that often indicates silent compression fractures in your spine. Developing a **stooped**

posture or **chronic back pain** can also mask small, unrecognized fractures that have already occurred.

Looking back, I had some of these warning signs. I'd noticed that my grip strength wasn't what it used to be, and my dentist had remarked that my gums were receding a bit. But like most people, I attributed these changes to "normal aging" rather than recognizing them as potential red flags for bone problems.

WHAT ACTUALLY HAPPENS DURING YOUR SCAN

Despite its intimidating name (dual-energy X-ray absorptiometry), a DEXA scan is remarkably simple and painless. The entire process takes about 15 minutes, involves less radiation than you'd get on a cross-country flight, and requires nothing more than lying still on a padded table.

You'll lie flat while a scanner arm passes quietly overhead, measuring bone density in your hip, your spine, and, sometimes, your forearm. Each site tells a different story about your bone health. Hip measurements are essential, because hip fractures are the ones most likely to steal your independence. Spine measurements can predict the risk of fractures that are often silent but can be deeply disabling over time. Forearm scans are used when arthritis or previous surgery makes the other sites unreliable.

The technician might position foam blocks under your knees or ask you to place your legs in a specific holder. This isn't uncomfortable, just necessary for getting accurate measurements. You'll need to remove any metal objects like jewelry or belts, but you can keep your clothes on. If the technician gives you specific instructions ("Hold still," "Don't cross your ankles," "Keep your arms at your sides"), follow them carefully. These aren't arbitrary requests; even small shifts in positioning can change your results enough to matter.

I wish I'd known all of this before my diagnosis. When I finally got my first DEXA scan (just after my fractures), I remember lying there thinking, "Why didn't I do this years ago?" The test was so quick and painless. If only I'd known what was brewing in my bones, maybe I could have prevented those fractures entirely.

THE IMPORTANCE OF A GOOD DEXA TECHNICIAN

That brings me to something I think deserves more attention: the person running your scan matters more than most people realize. You may have heard that DEXA scans are unreliable or inconsistent, and I understand why that perception exists. But the scan technology itself is highly precise. The real variability comes from the human side: how well the technician positions you, analyzes the scan, and maintains quality control.

Proper positioning is the single biggest factor in getting accurate, reproducible results. Organizations like the International Society for Clinical Densitometry (ISCD) and the American Registry of Radiologic Technologists (ARRT) offer specialized certifications in bone densitometry, but most states don't require them. In many facilities, a general radiology technician (without specific certification in bone density measurement) performs your DEXA scan as just one of many tasks in their day. That can be a problem, because when small differences in your numbers can determine whether a medication is recommended, started, or stopped, the quality of the scan isn't a minor detail. It's everything.

If you have the option, seek out facilities with densitometry-certified technicians; if possible, try to have the same technician perform your follow-up scans. Consistency in who runs the machine helps ensure that any changes in your numbers reflect real changes in your bones, not just differences in technique. If you can be tested on the exact same machine each time, too, that's even better.

MAKING SENSE OF YOUR NUMBERS

When I finally got my DEXA results after my fractures were discovered, the numbers told a story I hadn't expected. Your results center on two crucial scores that essentially answer the questions "How do your bones compare to the ideal?" and "How do they compare to others your age?"

But first, a quick word about what we're actually measuring.

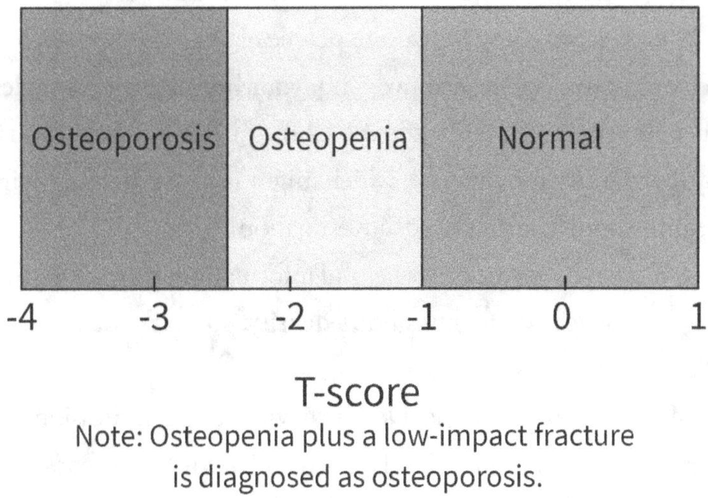

Figure 4.1: Understanding T-scores and their diagnostic categories.

Bone mineral density (BMD) is a measure of how tightly packed the minerals are in your bones. The denser the minerals, the stronger the bone. The scanner measures this for you but understanding what's behind the numbers helps you appreciate why the results matter and why the quality of the scan (and the technician performing it) is so important.

Your **T-score** compares your bone density to that of a healthy 30-year-old of your sex, effectively measuring how far you are from peak bone strength. Normal T-scores are –1.0 or higher. Osteopenia falls between –1.0 and –2.5. Osteoporosis gets diagnosed at –2.5 or lower.

Here's what those numbers mean in practical terms: each point on the scale represents a roughly 10–12% difference in bone density. So, a T-score of –2.5 means you have about 25% less bone than someone at peak density. That might not sound like much, but it represents a major increase in fracture risk.

Your **Z-score** compares you to people of your age, sex, and ethnicity. If your Z-score is above –2.0, your bone density is typical for your age group. A Z-score of –2.0 or below suggests unusually low density for your age, which might indicate an underlying medical condition that needs investigation.

While your Z-score offers helpful information, it's your T-score that most directly measures bone density, so that's the score I'll talk about the most.

My results surprised me. Despite having four compression fractures, my T-scores showed only osteopenia, not full osteoporosis. However, my doctor reminded me that the diagnosis isn't just about numbers, and that osteopenia plus fractures equals osteoporosis, regardless of what the T-score says. That taught me an important lesson: sometimes, your bones can break even when the numbers don't look terrible.

I'd been a doctor for decades, and I didn't fully understand how someone could fracture with "only" osteopenia. That's when I realized how much I (and probably many of my patients) had misunderstood bone fragility.

> **Did You Know?** More than half of all fragility fractures occur in people with osteopenia, not osteoporosis. Because so many more people have mild bone loss than severe, the majority of fractures happen in those whose T-scores don't look alarming.[19,20]

Sometimes, arthritis or surgical hardware can create false readings that make bones look denser than they really are, while other conditions might make them appear less dense. That's why having an experienced physician interpret your results is crucial; the numbers alone don't tell the whole story.

GOING BEYOND BASIC DENSITY NUMBERS

During my recovery, I learned that bone density tests don't tell the whole story. A T-score shows how strong your bones are right now, but it doesn't predict whether you're likely to break a bone in the future.

That's where a tool called the **Fracture Risk Assessment Tool (FRAX®)** comes in.[21] Instead of looking only at bone density, FRAX estimates your chance of breaking a bone over the next 10 years. FRAX isn't a test. Instead, it's a calculation that combines your bone density with other important factors such as your age, body mass index (BMI), family, smoking or alcohol use, steroid medications, and whether you've had a fracture before.

FRAX is often included in DEXA scan reports. Doctors often use it to help decide when treatment is needed. In the United States, treatment is commonly recommended if FRAX shows that the chance of a hip fracture is higher than 3%, or if the chance of a major fracture (like the spine, hip, or wrist) is higher than 20%, over the next 10 years. This is why fracture risk, not just the T-score, matters most.

However, FRAX isn't perfect. It doesn't fully capture some important details, like how recently a fracture occurred, how many fractures someone has had, or whether the individual is taking certain drugs (such as steroids) or has medical conditions that increase fracture risk (such as diabetes).

Researchers therefore developed **FRAXplus®**, an optional adjustment that allows medical providers to refine fracture risk estimates using additional information. This includes more details on things like recent fractures, falls, length of steroid use, and conditions such as diabetes. By considering these extra details, FRAXplus helps create a more personalized and realistic picture of fracture risk.

For me, FRAXplus showed that my fracture risk was double what regular FRAX predicted. This higher score was essential for convincing my insurance company to cover the expensive bone-building medication I needed. Unfortunately, not every doctor is familiar with this enhanced version of FRAX. More information for healthcare providers is available at fraxplus.org

The **trabecular bone score (TBS)** adds yet another layer by analyzing bone quality rather than just quantity. Remember that spongy bone at the core of your bones that we talked about in Chapter 3? Using the images from your DEXA scan, TBS examines the texture and strength of that inner honeycomb structure. Higher scores mean stronger, better-connected bone. Lower scores suggest the structure has weakened, which increases your fracture risk even if your bone density looks decent.

Conditions like diabetes, long-term steroid use, chronic inflammation, and other factors that I discuss in Chapter 6 can maintain reasonable bone density while degrading the internal structure (the fine honeycomb framework) that gives bones their strength. TBS reveals this hidden weakness that standard density measurements miss. My borderline-low TBS helped explain why I fractured despite my density numbers not looking terrible.

WHEN AND HOW OFTEN TO GET SCANNED

Most medical organizations recommend DEXA scanning for women at 65 and for men at 70 (or not at all), with earlier screening for those with risk factors. But after going through this experience, I think we should all have this test earlier. Ideally, you'd get your first scan in your 20s or 30s to establish your personal baseline before any decline begins.

One important clarification: if you've had your heel or wrist scanned at a health fair, pharmacy, or community screening event, that was not a DEXA scan. Those portable devices use ultrasound or small X-ray units to give a rough estimate of bone health, but they cannot diagnose osteoporosis, and their results cannot be directly compared to a central DEXA. If one of these screenings comes back low, take it as a "log in to your bank to check your balance" notice, not a bone bank statement itself. And even if the result looks fine, don't let it reassure you too much if you have risk factors. Follow up with a proper DEXA scan of your hip and spine to get the real numbers.

How often you need rescanning depends on your results and risk factors. Normal results might call for rechecking every 10–15 years, or at major hormonal transitions like menopause. Mild osteopenia suggests rescanning every five years, moderate osteopenia every three to five years, and advanced osteopenia every two years. If you have osteoporosis, you'll likely need annual monitoring.

Certain results require immediate, thorough evaluation. T-scores of –2.5 or lower at any site, Z-scores of –2.0 or below at any site, major drops since your last scan, or conflicting results between different skeletal sites all call for expert review.

TAKING CONTROL OF YOUR BONE HEALTH

Don't settle for vague reassurances like "Your bones are fine for your age" or "Don't worry about it yet." Ask for your exact T-scores and Z-scores. If the results seem borderline, ask about FRAXplus and TBS analysis. Remember that osteopenia combined with fractures constitutes osteoporosis, and push for a complete assessment if you have multiple risk factors.

Don't become obsessed with numbers; the goal is to have the information you need to make informed decisions about your bone health. Knowledge is power, and, in this case, it might be the power to prevent life-changing fractures.

As I studied my DEXA results during those long recovery months, the numbers told an important story about my bones. But numbers on a report can feel abstract. What isn't abstract is the impact fractures have on real lives: the pain, the lost independence, the fear of it happening again. Understanding the different types of osteoporotic fractures and how they happen (all of which we look at in the next chapter) became essential knowledge that I wish I'd had before my own diagnosis.

KEY TAKEAWAYS

- A DEXA scan is the gold standard for measuring bone density. T-scores of –2.5 or lower indicate osteoporosis, while T-scores between –1.0 and –2.5 indicate osteopenia.
- More than 54 million Americans over 50 have osteopenia or osteoporosis, and most of them don't know about it until a fracture occurs.
- Don't settle for vague reassurances; ask for your exact T-scores and Z-scores. If you have multiple risk factors, request FRAXplus and TBS analysis for a complete picture.

CHAPTER 5

UNDERSTANDING COMMON OSTEOPOROTIC FRACTURES

Vertebral, Hip, and Other Key Fractures

Learning about my four compression fractures was just the beginning of my journey to better understand how osteoporosis affects the skeleton. As I continued to research during my recovery, I realized that having knowledge about different types of fractures could help me recognize future problems early and understand what recovery might involve for each type. After all, T-scores are just numbers on a report. It's fractures that impact our well-being and our lives, and it's fractures that we're trying to avoid.

In this chapter, we'll walk through the most common osteoporotic fractures: vertebral, hip, and wrist. For each one, I'll cover what they feel like, how they're treated, and what recovery really looks like. I'll also share some difficult statistics on how these fractures affect quality of life and, in some cases, survival. Those numbers deserve context, and, as we'll see, they're more nuanced than they first appear.

Osteoporotic fractures, or "fragility fractures," differ dramatically from the broken bones that result from major trauma like car accidents or sports injuries. They occur from minimal impact or what doctors call "low-energy trauma," such as falls from standing height (like tripping over a curb), minor bumps, or sometimes even routine activities like coughing or bending over. Understanding this difference helped me recognize how serious my condition really was.

WHAT THE SCARY STATISTICS REALLY MEAN

Before we start exploring specific fracture types, I need to be honest with you: some of the statistics in this chapter are frightening. When my early readers first saw the numbers on death and disability after fractures, they pushed back. "Are people really dying because of the fracture," they asked, "or were they already sicker to begin with?"

The answer is that two things are true at once. Fractures happen more often in sicker people, *and* fractures make people sicker. Understanding how both of these truths work together turns a scary number into something far more useful and far more empowering.

Fractures happen more in sicker people.

The people who sustain fragility fractures tend to already be more vulnerable than their peers. They may have lower bone density, weaker muscles, balance problems, or chronic conditions like heart disease, diabetes, dementia, or kidney disease. These underlying problems were already increasing their risk of dying; the fracture just made those problems more visible. In studies that take these background health factors into account, a large share of the higher death rates seen after a fracture can be attributed to reasons other than bone loss. The fracture was, in part, a signal of trouble that was already brewing.

And fractures make people sicker.

A hip fracture may mean such serious things as emergency surgery, immobility, blood clots, pneumonia, and rapid muscle loss. Meanwhile, vertebral fractures can produce pain that limits movement, progressive spinal deformity that can compromise breathing, and a cascade of additional fractures. Even after carefully matching fracture patients to similar people who didn't fracture (same age, same health conditions, same functional level), people with fractures still have significantly higher mortality rates, especially in the first three to six months. In some analyses, roughly one-third to one-half of the extra deaths in the first year after a hip fracture can be traced directly to the fracture and its complications, not to pre-existing illness alone.

Why does this matter for you? Because the damage caused by the fracture itself and its aftermath, the part where fractures make people sicker, is exactly where your actions and your care team's actions can make the biggest difference. You can't change your age, and you may not be able to erase all your health conditions. But you can push for timely surgery and coordinated care. You can get out of bed and get moving early. You can start bone-strengthening treatment. You can invest in rehabilitation. These aren't empty reassurances; they're backed by data that I'll share with you throughout this chapter.

Keep this in mind as we look at specific fracture types. When you encounter a sobering statistic, remember: part of that number reflects health problems that existed before the break, and part reflects the fracture itself. And that second part is where you have real power to change the outcome.

VERTEBRAL COMPRESSION FRACTURES: THE SILENT EPIDEMIC

Vertebral compression fractures are the most common osteoporotic fractures, affecting approximately 700,000 to 1.5 million Americans annually. They occur when weakened vertebrae can no longer support normal loads and thus collapse, typically crushing into a wedge shape.[22]

What shocked me during my research was learning how these fractures often happen. Unlike dramatic back injuries from major accidents, compression fractures frequently occur during the most mundane activities. Bending forward to pick up groceries, lifting a small child, coughing forcefully during illness, or even getting out of bed can trigger these fractures in people with severely weakened bones.

My own fractures happened during what seemed like a minor fall, but I now understand that my bones had probably been on the verge of fracturing for some time. The fall with Finnegan was simply the final straw.

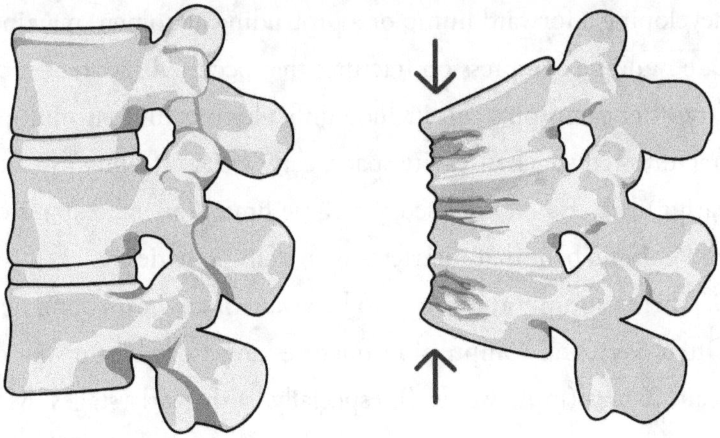

Figure 5.1: Vertebral compression fracture. The arrows show the compressive forces that cause a weakened vertebra to collapse into a wedge shape, which can lead to height loss and spinal curvature.

Recognizing the Warning Signs

Sudden onset of severe back pain is the most common symptom, often described as sharp, stabbing, or crushing pain that worsens with movement. Many report that the pain is worst when standing or walking and least when lying on their side. Interestingly, not all compression fractures cause immediate severe pain or even much pain at all. Some develop gradually with only mild discomfort, which people attribute to muscle strain or arthritis.

Height loss can be a subtle but important sign. Losing more than 1.5 inches from your peak adult height or 0.8 inches in a single year warrants investigation. Changes in posture, including developing a forward hump or a protruding abdomen, may indicate multiple compression fractures that occurred silently.

Other symptoms can include difficulty breathing if multiple fractures reduce chest cavity space, early satiety (feeling full after eating) because compressed vertebrae limit stomach expansion, and chronic pain that interferes with daily activities.

There's an important note to be aware of about imaging here. Often, vertebral compression fractures aren't picked up well on plain X-rays (mine weren't!), especially in the early stages. MRI is much more sensitive; it can reveal not only the deformity but also the swelling and fluid inside the bones that indicate a fresh fracture. Don't be afraid to ask for an MRI if you have persistent midline back pain, especially if it came on after a fall and you have risk factors for osteoporosis.

Treatment and Recovery Reality

My recovery from compression fractures taught me that the healing process is often longer and more complex than people expect. Acute compression fractures typically require 6–12 weeks to heal; multiple fractures can take a year or more. Treatment focuses on pain management, maintaining function, and preventing additional fractures.

The shoulder-to-hip back brace I had to wear was hot, uncomfortable, and a constant reminder of my fragility. It was definitely not flattering or attractive. But it provided necessary support during healing while my bones knitted back together. Physical therapy helped me maintain my mobility and strengthen the surrounding muscles once the acute pain subsided.

If vertebral fractures are diagnosed early enough, procedures like vertebroplasty or kyphoplasty can provide relief by injecting bone cement into the collapsed vertebra. While these procedures can stabilize the bones and relieve pain, they also have risks: in rare cases, the cement can leak and press on the spinal cord and, very rarely, cause numbness or even paralysis. It's also possible that another fracture will later develop above or below the treated vertebrae, as the forces on the adjacent bones change with the additional mass from the cement. Regardless of whether you undergo a procedure, the most critical aspect of treatment involves preventing additional fractures through aggressive osteoporosis management.

A Note About Silent Vertebral Fractures

If you're told that there are old compression fractures in your spine that you never knew you had, you aren't alone. Many people first learn they've had compression fractures when X-rays or computed tomography (CT) scans are ordered for other conditions. While it's shocking, at least your fractures didn't cause you pain! It's not clear why these fractures can be very painful or not painful at all. Also, please be aware that even if your fractures were silent, you may still be at substantial risk for other fractures.

The Real Impact of Vertebral Fractures

When I was recovering from my four compression fractures, people would sometimes say things like, "At least it's not a hip fracture." I understood what they meant. They were trying to be reassuring, as most people know how life-changing a hip fracture can be. But the more I researched, the more I realized that vertebral fractures carry their own serious consequences that deserve honest conversation. They aren't minor injuries, and dismissing them as "just" back problems does a disservice to anyone living through the pain, the limitations, and the fear that follows.

Mortality After Vertebral Fractures

Vertebral fractures don't carry the same dramatic mortality statistics as hip fractures, but they do increase the risk of dying. Large population studies show that people who sustain an osteoporotic vertebral fracture have about a 1.5–2 times higher risk of death over the following 5–10 years (with the highest risk in the first year) compared to similar people who haven't fractured. One-year mortality rates are generally in the range of 7–9%: lower than hip fractures but clearly elevated above what you'd expect for someone of the same age and health status.[23,24]

In some older, sicker populations, the numbers are higher. One study found one-year death rates for vertebral fractures approaching 28% in patients in their 80s and beyond, likely because these patients had more underlying health problems to begin with. Remember, both truths apply here: vertebral fractures happen more often in people who are already unwell, *and* vertebral fractures make people sicker through pain, immobility, spinal deformity, and breathing problems. In younger adults, when researchers account for background health factors, much of the increased risk of dying shrinks considerably. In older adults and men, a meaningful portion of that risk persists even after that accounting, which is evidence that the fracture itself is doing real harm.

Multiple Fractures Multiply the Risk

This is something that unfortunately applied directly to me with my four fractures. Research consistently shows a dose–response relationship: the more vertebrae that fracture, the higher the mortality risk. Repeated vertebral fractures can keep mortality elevated for up to a decade. Each additional broken vertebra compounds not just the pain and deformity but also the potential breathing problems, the loss of mobility, and the risk of dying.

Think of it this way: one compression fracture is a serious warning. Multiple compression fractures represent cumulative damage to your body's core structure, and the risks rise with each additional fracture.

Quality of Life: The Impact You Live With

Beyond mortality, vertebral fractures take a significant toll on daily life, and this is something I can speak to personally. Studies comparing people with vertebral fractures to age-matched peers consistently find worse scores in mobility, self-care, ability to do usual activities, pain levels, and anxiety and depression. These aren't small differences. On standard quality of life scales, vertebral fracture patients show clinically meaningful drops that often persist well beyond the first year.

Vertebral fractures often strike people in their 50s, 60s, and 70s, years when many expect to remain fully active. The chronic back pain, the height loss, the changes in posture, the difficulty standing for long periods or carrying things: these affect everything from traveling to playing with grandchildren to simply feeling like yourself. I remember the frustration of not being able to load the dishwasher without pain, of watching my posture change in the mirror, and of worrying whether every twinge meant another fracture.

Multiple and more severe fractures make all of this worse. If you've had two or more compression fractures, research shows significantly greater disability and lower quality of life than if you'd had just one.

FIVE WAYS TO PROTECT YOUR QUALITY OF LIFE AFTER A VERTEBRAL FRACTURE

Vertebral fractures often arrive earlier than hip fractures, but they're not minor. If you've had one, taking these steps can meaningfully change your trajectory.

1. Treat pain so you can move, not so you can stay in bed. Untreated pain leads to lying still, weaker muscles, more stiffness, and a higher risk of additional fractures. Work with your clinicians on a pain plan (medications, bracing, heat, or sometimes nerve-targeted treatments) that keeps the pain tolerable enough for you to stand and walk safely.

2. Start bone-strengthening treatment after the first fracture. A vertebral fracture is a loud warning about bone strength. People who start osteoporosis medications after a fragility fracture have fewer new fractures and, in some studies, 20–30% lower mortality over the following two to five years than those who go untreated. Ask your clinician about options, and make sure you're getting adequate vitamin D and calcium.[25]

3. Work on posture, back strength, and balance.

Back extensor and core-strengthening exercises, ideally taught by a physical therapist, can reduce pain, improve posture, and make everyday activities easier after a compression fracture. Gentle balance and strength training also lower your chances of another fall and another fracture.

4. Don't ignore your mood, fear of movement, or social withdrawal.

Many people with vertebral fractures develop chronic worry about falling, low mood, or loss of confidence, which in turn makes their quality of life even worse. Tell your clinicians if you feel afraid to move, down, or isolated. Reassurance, graded activity plans, counseling, or medications when needed can help you stay engaged with life.

5. Take steps now to avoid a "cascade" of new fractures.

Each additional broken vertebra compounds pain, deformity, breathing problems, disability, and risk of early death. Beyond medication, reduce that risk by reviewing your medications for drugs that increase the risk of falling, making your home safer (lighting, rugs, stairs, grab bars, footwear), and maintaining muscle with regular safe activity and enough protein in your diet.

HIP FRACTURES: THE LIFE-CHANGER

Hip fractures are the most serious osteoporotic fractures, with significant impacts on independence, quality of life, and even survival.

Nearly 300,000 Americans over 65 are hospitalized for hip fractures each year, with the vast majority of those fractures related to osteoporosis.[26]

Most hip fractures result from falls, particularly sideways falls that impact the hip directly. However, people with severe osteoporosis can sustain hip fractures from minimal trauma, like stepping off a curb awkwardly or even rotating while standing.

Hip fractures almost always require surgical repair, typically within 24–48 hours of injury. The type of surgery depends on the fracture location and bone quality. Recovery involves early mobilization, because people must get up and moving right away after surgery to prevent complications like blood clots and pneumonia.

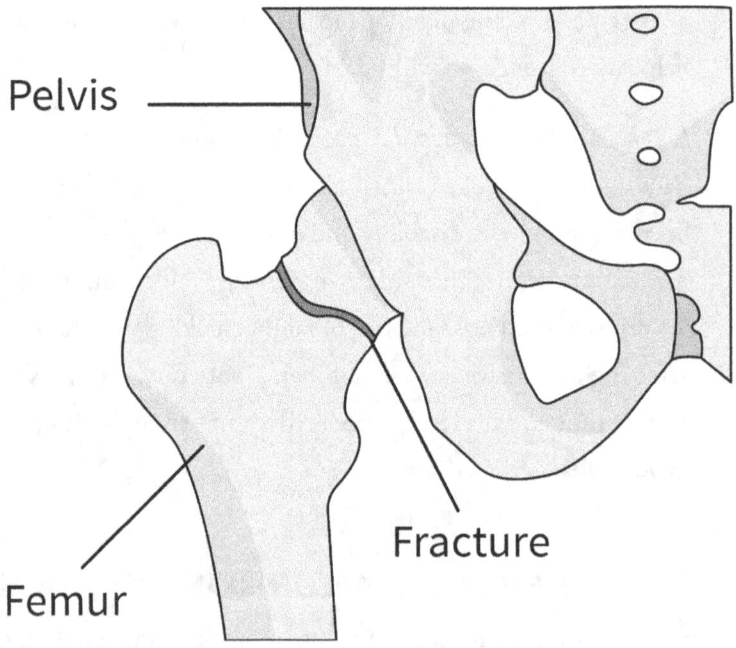

Figure 5.2: Hip fracture occurring at the femoral neck, the most common location for osteoporotic hip fractures.

The statistics surrounding hip fracture recovery are sobering. Studies show one-year mortality rates generally ranging from 15% to 25%, though rates above 30% have been reported in older, sicker populations, and only about 40–60% of survivors return to their prior level of independence. Men face even higher mortality rates after hip fractures, with studies showing death rates of up to 37% within the first year. This is partly because men tend to be older at diagnosis, more often have other serious medical conditions, and often experience delays in diagnosis and treatment. However, these grim statistics don't apply equally to all patients: younger, healthier individuals with better bone quality often recover more completely.[27,28,29]

Did You Know? The most effective osteoporosis medications can reduce hip fracture risk by 40–50% in high-risk patients. In large clinical trials, people who started and continued treatment had significantly lower odds of breaking a hip. These are more than just numbers; they represent maintained independence, avoided surgeries, and a life lived on your own terms.[30],[31]

The Real Impact of Hip Fractures: What Those Numbers Really Mean

I know those mortality statistics are hard to read. But remember what we discussed earlier in this chapter: fractures happen more often in sicker people, *and* fractures make people sicker.

Understanding how those two truths play out with hip fractures, and how the numbers vary by age and sex, gives you something more useful than fear: a clearer sense of where action matters most.

Age and Sex Matter More Than You Might Think

The often-quoted "20–30% mortality" figure is a population average, and it masks enormous variation depending on who you are and how healthy you were before the fracture.

Consider this: among women in their late 60s, roughly one out of 100 would typically die in a given year from all causes. If all those women sustained a hip fracture, about six or seven out of 100 would die within the year. That's a four- to five-fold increase, which is alarming in relative terms but still means that the large majority would survive and recover. For women in their 80s and beyond, the background risk is already higher, and one-year mortality after a hip fracture often reaches 15–25%.

Men consistently fare worse. At every age, men have higher death rates after a hip fracture than women, often by 5–10 percentage points. In some studies, men in their 80s have one-year death rates above 25% after a hip fracture. This likely reflects a combination of higher rates of other serious health conditions in men who fracture, less physical resilience and ability to bounce back, and, sometimes, delays in recognizing osteoporosis in men in the first place.

The bottom line: your individual risk depends heavily on your age, sex, and overall health going into the fracture. A relatively healthy 65-year-old woman who breaks a hip has a very different outlook from an 85-year-old man with heart disease and diabetes.

Where Action Makes the Difference

Here's the good news: the portion of hip fracture mortality where the fracture makes people sicker (through surgery complications, immobility, blood clots, pneumonia, and deconditioning) is concentrated in the first three to six months. And that's exactly where good care and early action have the most power. Research on early mobilization, coordinated geriatric–orthopedic care, and aggressive management of other medical conditions shows meaningful reductions in complications and death.

Your age isn't something you can change, and it may not be possible to fully address all of your health conditions. But if you or someone you love breaks a hip, the following steps can genuinely tilt the odds.

FIVE WAYS TO PROTECT YOUR QUALITY OF LIFE AFTER A HIP FRACTURE

Hip fractures happen more often in people who are already vulnerable, and hip fractures make people sicker. You can't eliminate the extra risk entirely, but these steps can meaningfully lower it and improve both survival and independence.

1. Start moving as soon as it's safely possible to do so.
Staying in bed too long after surgery is a major reason people lose independence, develop complications, and never get back to their prior level of walking. Ask your care team, "When can I safely get out of bed, stand, and take a few steps with help?" Aim to move a little every day.

2. Take rehabilitation seriously. This is your "job" for the year.

People who work consistently with physical and occupational therapists, first in the hospital and then in rehab or at home, are more likely to walk again, manage daily tasks, and report better quality of life a year later. Treat therapy sessions like essential appointments, not optional extras.

3. Protect your mood, not just your hip.

Depression, anxiety, and fear of falling after a fracture strongly predict who will struggle the most with pain and independence. Tell your doctor if you feel down or hopeless, and ask about counseling, support groups, or medications if needed. Emotional recovery is part of physical recovery.

4. Review your medications and fall risks.

Certain medications (like strong sleeping pills, sedatives, or blood pressure pills that drop your blood pressure too low) can worsen dizziness and falls, which erode quality of life. After a hip fracture, ask for a full medication review and a home fall risk check that includes lighting, rugs, stairs, footwear, grab bars, and assistive devices.

5. Feed your bones and muscles.

Healing a broken hip is like training for a marathon: your body needs fuel and building blocks. Poor appetite, low protein intake, and weak muscles are all linked to worse outcomes after hip fracture. Aim for regular meals with protein at each one (if your kidneys allow), stay hydrated, and ask for a dietitian or nutrition consultation as part of your recovery plan.

OTHER FRACTURES WORTH KNOWING ABOUT

Vertebral and hip fractures get most of the attention in osteoporosis conversations, and for good reason. But they aren't the only fractures that weak bones can cause. A few other fracture types deserve your awareness, both because some of them serve as early warnings that your bones need help and because others can be surprisingly difficult to diagnose.

Wrist, Rib, and Upper Arm Fractures: The Early Warnings

Wrist fractures often serve as the first sign of underlying bone loss, typically occurring 10–15 years before hip fractures. They usually result from falling forward and instinctively extending your arms to break the fall. Rib fractures, especially multiple rib fractures after a simple fall from standing, are another sign of weakening bones.

Upper arm fractures near the shoulder (what doctors call "proximal humerus fractures") are the third most common osteoporotic fracture after vertebral and wrist fractures, but they rarely get mentioned in patient-facing discussions about osteoporosis. About 85% occur in those over 50, and the incidence peaks between people's 60s and 80s, with women affected roughly two to four times as often as men. Like wrist fractures, they typically happen after a fall onto an outstretched hand or directly onto the shoulder. Most are treated without surgery using a sling and physical therapy, though more complex breaks may require surgical repair.[32]

What makes wrist, rib, and upper arm fractures so important isn't their severity (most heal well and don't typically cause long-term disability) but what they signal. These fractures are your skeleton's early alarm system. They're telling you that your bones are weaker than they should be, and that without intervention, more serious fractures could follow. If you break a wrist, a rib, or your upper arm after a simple fall, don't make the mistake of thinking, "It's just a wrist" or "Plenty of healthy people crack a rib." Ask your healthcare provider to order a DEXA scan. That conversation could prevent a vertebral or hip fracture down the road.

Pelvic Fractures: The Underrecognized Threat

Pelvic "insufficiency" fractures are increasingly common in older adults with osteoporosis, but they remain underrecognized, partly because they can be surprisingly hard to diagnose. These fractures account for an estimated 5–8% of all osteoporosis-related fractures, and their incidence has risen sharply over recent decades as the population ages.

What makes pelvic fractures tricky is that they often don't show up on standard X-rays. Pain in the lower back, buttocks, or groin after a fall (or sometimes with no clear injury at all) can easily be attributed to muscle strain or arthritis. Diagnosis often requires a CT or MRI. If you have osteoporosis and develop persistent pain in your lower back, pelvis, or groin that doesn't improve with rest, push for advanced imaging rather than accepting a vague diagnosis.

Pelvic fractures are not early warning fractures. They tend to occur in people in their 70s and beyond, in the same age group and health profile as hip fractures. And like hip fractures, they can cause significant pain, prolonged immobility, loss of independence, and mortality rates that approach those of hip fractures. They deserve to be taken just as seriously.

RECOGNITION AND RESPONSE

Understanding common fracture patterns helps you recognize potential problems early and seek proper treatment. Severe back pain that develops suddenly, particularly after any jarring movement, may indicate a compression fracture. Inability to bear weight after a fall suggests a possible hip or pelvic fracture.

More concerning symptoms include numbness or tingling in the legs after a back injury, which could indicate spinal cord involvement, or severe breathing difficulty after chest trauma, which might suggest multiple rib fractures. These require immediate emergency medical attention.

THE CASCADE EFFECT

One of the most concerning aspects of osteoporotic fractures is the cascade effect: how one fracture dramatically increases the risk of additional fractures. People who experience one vertebral compression fracture have a five-fold increased risk of additional spinal fractures and a two-to-three-fold increased risk of a hip fracture.[33]

This cascade occurs partly because structural changes from one fracture alter loading patterns throughout the skeleton, placing additional stress on other bones. Additionally, the activity restriction and muscle weakness that often follow fractures can accelerate bone loss and increase fall risk.

Understanding this cascade effect motivated me to take my

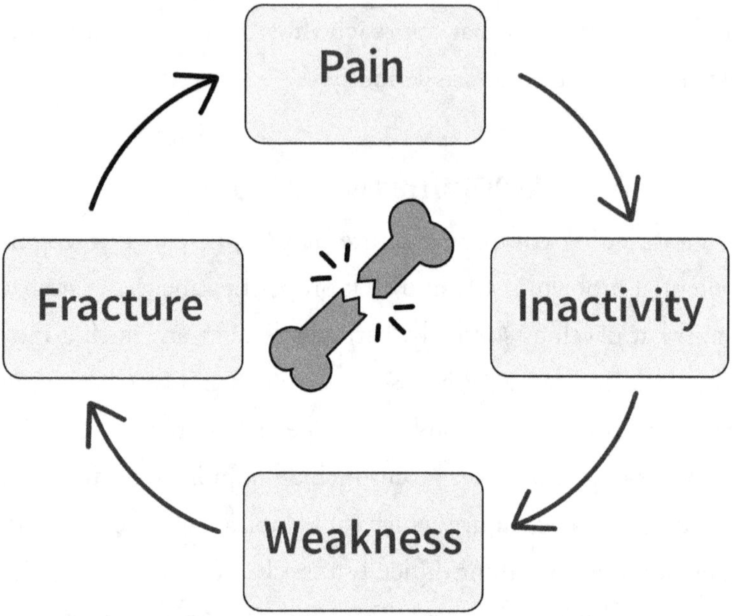

Figure 5.3: Fracture pain can lead to inactivity and weakness, leading to another fracture.

treatment seriously. Preventing the fifth fracture became just as important as recovering from the first four.

LIVING AFTER FRACTURE

Experiencing osteoporotic fractures doesn't mean your active life is over, but it does require adjustments and increased vigilance. Most people, me included, can recover well from fractures and continue to live independently with appropriate precautions and treatment.

The key involves balancing reasonable caution with continued engagement in life. Completely avoiding activity often leads to further bone loss and muscle weakness, increasing future fracture risk. Instead, I focused on modifying risky activities while maintaining safe exercise and social engagement.

Recovery from osteoporotic fractures often takes longer than expected and requires patience with the healing process. However, many people find that the experience motivates them to take better care of their bone health and overall fitness, leading to improvements in areas they hadn't previously addressed.

HOPE FOR THE FUTURE

While learning about osteoporotic fractures can feel overwhelming, remember that knowledge is power. Understanding these risks helps guide prevention efforts that may help you avoid these complications entirely. The goal isn't to live in fear of fractures but to live wisely, with awareness of the risks and confidence in your ability to manage them effectively.

Effective treatments exist for osteoporosis, and research continues to develop new approaches for both prevention and treatment. With proper medical care and reasonable safety precautions, many people with osteoporosis continue to live active, independent lives.

My own journey from those four compression fractures to renewed strength and confidence proves that osteoporotic fractures, while serious, don't have to define or limit your future. With the right knowledge and support, you can move forward with hope and determination toward a stronger, healthier future.

But understanding fractures raised a deeper question for me: what had caused my bones to weaken so dramatically in the first place? The fall with Finnegan was the final straw, but the weakness had been building for years. The more I researched, the more I uncovered factors that had been quietly undermining my bones while I went about my busy life, completely unaware. And that's exactly what we'll explore in Chapter 6.

KEY TAKEAWAYS

- Fractures happen more often in sicker people, and fractures make people sicker. Understanding both truths helps you focus on the factors you can actually control.
- Hip fractures have the most profound consequences: only 40–60% of patients return to their previous level of independence, and one-year mortality ranges from about 7% in younger women to over 25% in older men.
- After any osteoporotic fracture, taking action (early mobilization, bone-strengthening treatment, rehabilitation, mood support, and fall prevention) can meaningfully improve both survival and quality of life.

CHAPTER 6

THE HIDDEN THIEVES

How Unseen Factors Affect Bone Health

Not all threats to bone health announce themselves loudly. Some work quietly in the background, slowly eroding strength over months or years while you stay completely unaware. During my recovery research, I started thinking of these as "hidden thieves": factors that steal bone health while we go about our daily lives, oblivious to the damage being done.

Understanding these thieves was both enlightening and frustrating. Enlightening because it helped explain how I'd ended up with four compression fractures at 55. Frustrating because some of these factors had been affecting my bones for years, and despite all my medical knowledge, I hadn't paid attention and connected the dots.

THE UNAVOIDABLE CULPRITS

Some bone thieves simply come with the territory of being human. Age tops the list, and there's no getting around it. As the decades accumulate, bone remodeling gradually shifts toward more withdrawals than deposits. We can slow this process, but we can't stop it entirely. I had to accept that my 55-year-old bones weren't going to behave like my 25-year-old bones, no matter what I did.

Hormonal changes hit women particularly hard. Estrogen helps keep the peace between bone-building and bone-removing cells, so when levels plummet at menopause, the balance tips dramatically toward bone loss.

I'd gone through early menopause after a hysterectomy at 47, which meant I'd been without estrogen's protection for eight years before my fractures. Looking back, this should have been a huge red flag for bone health monitoring. But like many women, I was focused on managing hot flashes and mood changes, not thinking about what was happening to my skeleton.

FAMILY HISTORY: THE CARDS YOU'RE DEALT

Genetics load the dice when it comes to osteoporosis risk. If your mother or grandmother had a "dowager's hump" (a hunched-over back) or broke a hip, that information matters more than you might think. Family history affects everything from your peak bone mass to how quickly you lose bone as you age.

In my own case, I discovered that Ehlers–Danlos syndrome (EDS) runs in my family. This rare disorder affects the production of collagen, the protein that forms the framework for bone tissue. While my genetic tests were inconclusive, EDS is a known risk factor for osteoporosis because weak collagen leads to weak bones. This may have been another contributing factor to my fractures.

THE WEIGHT LOSS CONNECTION

Other thieves work more subtly, often going unrecognized for years. Rapid weight loss was one that surprised me, and it hit close to home. In the two years before my fractures, I'd lost about 50 pounds, which seemed like a good thing at the time. However, I now realize I lost considerable muscle mass along with the weight, because I didn't include enough exercise in my weight loss plan.

While losing excess weight is generally healthy, dramatic weight loss (especially when it includes considerable muscle loss) removes the mechanical stress that tells bones to stay strong. Having a very low body weight (BMI under 18.5) or a history of anorexia is also a risk for osteoporosis. If a special diet or a new weight loss medicine is helping you lose weight, don't forget to protect your bones. Get enough protein and calcium, and, most importantly, get regular weight-bearing exercise to preserve your muscles and skeleton.

WHEN MEDICATIONS BECOME BONE THIEVES

Medications that can quietly undermine bone health were a real eye-opener for me as a physician. I'd prescribed many of these medications over the years without always fully considering their long-term bone health implications. Some medications are prescribed to help serious conditions, but they can have unintended effects on your skeleton.

Corticosteroids and Inflammation Fighters

Corticosteroids (medicines like prednisone that reduce inflammation) top this list. Even multiple short courses of prednisone for severe asthma or poison ivy can affect bones, while long-term use for conditions like rheumatoid arthritis or inflammatory bowel disease can cause dramatic bone loss that often begins within the first few months of treatment.[34],[35]

Did You Know? Corticosteroids cause bone loss in two phases: a rapid initial loss of 6–12% in the first year, followed by a slower decline of about 3% annually. Even low doses of prednisone can cause measurable bone damage within just weeks of starting treatment.[36,37]

Cancer Treatment Medications

Cancer treatments create another major category of medication-related bone loss. Aromatase inhibitors for breast cancer eliminate estrogen's protective effects, often causing bone loss in women that exceeds that seen with natural menopause. Androgen deprivation therapy for prostate cancer does the same thing to men's bones by eliminating testosterone.

If you're facing cancer treatment, it's crucial to ask your oncologist whether any specific measures should be taken to support your bone health before, during, or after treatment. Many cancer centers now have protocols for bone health monitoring and protection during treatments known to affect bones, but these can sometimes be overlooked during the difficult days of cancer treatment.

Injectable Birth Control Medication

Depo-Provera (medroxyprogesterone acetate) is an injectable hormonal contraceptive given every three months. You may know this as the "birth control shot." It carries a U.S. Food and Drug Administration (FDA) black box warning for significant bone mineral density loss with long-term use (a "black box warning" is a high-level warning for serious drug risk). It works by suppressing estrogen; this means it removes the same bone-protective effect that disappears at menopause, just earlier in life. Women who have used Depo-Provera for birth control should ask their doctor whether their bone health should be assessed.

The SSRI and Antidepressant Story

One category I hadn't previously associated with bone health was antidepressants, and particularly a type called selective serotonin reuptake inhibitors (SSRIs): medications like fluoxetine, sertraline, and paroxetine. These medications are incredibly common; about 13% of American adults take antidepressants, and the percentage is even higher in women over 60. Given how widespread their use is, even a modest increase in fracture risk affects a lot of people.[38]

Some studies show that SSRIs are associated with increased fracture risk, especially at higher doses or with long-term use. The exact reason isn't clear, but researchers think SSRIs may interfere with how bones rebuild themselves. The mechanism is still debated, partly because depression itself can also affect bone health through reduced activity, poor nutrition, and elevated stress hormones; this makes it difficult to fully untangle the drug's contribution from the condition these medicines treat.[39,40,41]

A Critical Note About Stopping Mental Health Medications

Depression and anxiety are serious medical conditions, and,

for many people, the benefits of effective mental healthcare still outweigh possible bone risks. If you're taking SSRIs or serotonin–norepinephrine reuptake inhibitors (SNRIs), a related type of antidepressant, do *not* stop them without the guidance of your healthcare provider.

The goal is simply to be aware that these commonly prescribed medications may quietly influence bone health over long periods of time. By understanding this connection, you and your doctor can make informed decisions and take proactive steps to protect your bones, whether that means earlier screening, lifestyle adjustments, or simply a more tailored risk assessment for osteoporosis.

Other Common Medications That Affect Bones

Several other medications can quietly weaken bones: certain anti-seizure drugs, excessive thyroid hormone replacement (doses higher than the body needs), and even proton pump inhibitors for acid reflux when used for extended periods.

UNDERSTANDING YOUR MEDICATION RISK: A QUICK REFERENCE

Here's a guide to medications that may affect bone health. This list isn't exhaustive, and the presence of a medication here *does not mean* you should stop taking it. What's important is being aware of the potential bone effects, so you and your healthcare team can use appropriate monitoring (DEXA scans; see Chapter 4) and protective strategies (exercise and diet; see Chapters 7 and 8, respectively).

Medication Category	Examples	What to Know
Glucocorticoids/ corticosteroids	Prednisone (Deltasone), methylprednisolone (Medrol), dexamethasone (Decadron)	Even short courses can affect bones; long-term use causes dramatic bone loss
Aromatase inhibitors	Anastrozole (Arimidex), letrozole (Femara), exemestane (Aromasin)	Used for breast cancer; eliminate estrogen's bone protection
Androgen deprivation therapy	Leuprolide (Lupron), goserelin (Zoladex), degarelix (Firmagon)	Used for prostate cancer; eliminate testosterone's bone protection
Hormonal contraceptives (injectable)	Medroxyprogesterone (Depo-Provera)	FDA black box warning for bone loss; greatest risk with long-term use
SSRIs	Fluoxetine, sertraline, paroxetine, citalopram, escitalopram	Risk may increase with duration, especially after 5+ years
SNRIs	Venlafaxine, duloxetine	Similar possible risks to SSRIs
Anti-seizure medications	Phenytoin (Dilantin), carbamazepine (Tegretol), phenobarbital (Luminal), valproic acid (Depakote)	Enzyme-inducing drugs particularly affect bone metabolism
Proton pump inhibitors	Omeprazole, esomeprazole, lansoprazole, pantoprazole	Risk increases with long-term use (years, not months)
Excess thyroid hormone	Levothyroxine (Synthroid, Levoxyl) over-treatment	Too much accelerates bone turnover
Thiazolidinediones	Pioglitazone (Actos), rosiglitazone (for diabetes)	May increase fracture risk, particularly in women
Loop diuretics	Furosemide (Lasix)	May affect calcium excretion
Anticoagulants	Heparin (with long-term use)	Long-term use may affect bone
Methotrexate	High-dose or long-term use	May affect bone with extended use

Medication Category	Examples	What to Know
Calcineurin inhibitors	Cyclosporine, tacrolimus (transplant medications)	Used after organ transplants; multiple mechanisms affect bone
Some antipsychotics	Various	May work through effects on a hormone called prolactin

WHEN CHRONIC ILLNESS STEALS BONE STRENGTH

It's not just medications that can cause problems for your bone bank. Chronic illness can quietly sap the strength of your skeleton. They often steal bone strength in multiple ways, creating a perfect storm of bone loss.

Rheumatoid Arthritis and Inflammatory Diseases

Rheumatoid arthritis (RA) is a particularly strong risk factor for osteoporosis: the chronic inflammation that characterizes the condition directly damages bone tissue, while the medications used to treat it (especially corticosteroids) compound the problem. The inflammatory process in RA stimulates bone breakdown while suppressing bone formation in a double assault on skeletal strength.

Other inflammatory diseases, like lupus and Crohn's disease, create similar problems, requiring steroid treatment that further accelerates bone loss.

Celiac Disease: The Hidden Malabsorption Problem

Celiac disease was particularly interesting to research: we think of celiac disease, a severe reaction to gluten in the diet, as a problem of the bowels, not the bones. Yet many people with undiagnosed celiac have serious bone loss, because their damaged intestines can't properly absorb calcium, vitamin D, and other bone-building nutrients, even when their diet appears adequate. The inflammation from untreated celiac also directly harms bone tissue.

Thyroid and Parathyroid Problems

Overactive thyroid conditions accelerate bone turnover dramatically. Imagine your bone remodeling process stuck in fast-forward mode. Even people taking too much thyroid hormone replacement medication can inadvertently damage their bones over time. If you're on thyroid medication, regular monitoring ensures your dose isn't higher than necessary.

But there's another gland that deserves attention: one that many people have never heard of until it causes problems.

Your parathyroid glands are four tiny structures, each about the size of a grain of rice, tucked behind your thyroid in your neck. Despite their small size, they play an enormous role in bone health. Their sole job is to regulate calcium levels in your blood by producing parathyroid hormone (PTH). When blood calcium levels

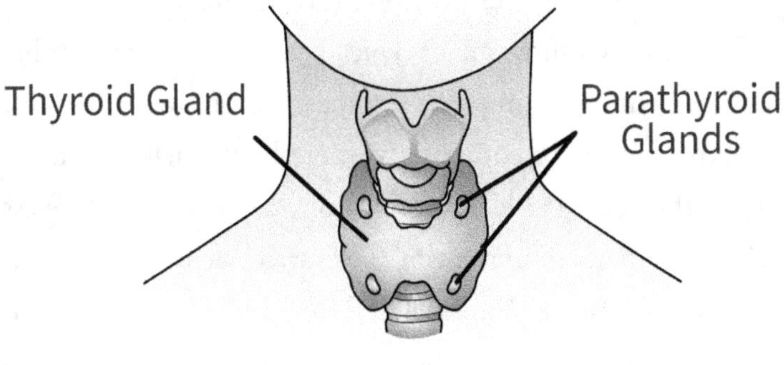

Figure 6.1: The location of the parathyroid glands.

drop, PTH signals your bones to release calcium, making a withdrawal from your bone bank.

In primary hyperparathyroidism, one or more of these glands becomes overactive, usually due to a small benign tumor called an adenoma. The gland keeps pumping out PTH even when calcium levels are already normal or high. The result? Your bones are constantly being told to release calcium, whether your body needs it or not. It's like having a bank teller who keeps withdrawing money from your account that you don't need, without your permission.

This condition is surprisingly common, affecting roughly one to seven in 1,000 adults. The highest rates (about one in 500) are in postmenopausal women: the same group already at elevated risk for osteoporosis. Many people with hyperparathyroidism have no obvious symptoms for years, though some experience fatigue, kidney stones, depression, or "brain fog." The bone loss, meanwhile, happens silently.[42]

The good news is that hyperparathyroidism is one of the few causes of osteoporosis that can be cured. If a parathyroid adenoma is identified, surgical removal is often straightforward (performed by an experienced surgeon, it's typically an outpatient procedure), and bone density can improve significantly afterward.

This is why your osteoporosis workup should include both a calcium level and a PTH level, not just one or the other. The classic finding in hyperparathyroidism is elevated calcium and elevated PTH together. That isn't normal; if the calcium level in your blood is high, it should signal the body to make less PTH. Don't hesitate to ask your doctor about these results specifically.

Cushing's Syndrome: When Your Body Makes Too Much Cortisol

Earlier in this chapter, I mentioned how corticosteroid medications like prednisone can damage bones. But your body can also overproduce cortisol (a natural form of steroid) on its own, and the effect on your skeleton is just as damaging. In Cushing's syndrome, your body churns out excess cortisol around the clock. This constant flood suppresses your bone-building osteoblasts while ramping up the osteoclasts that tear bone down, and it interferes with calcium absorption and vitamin D metabolism as well. Studies have found osteoporosis in 30 to 50% of people with Cushing's syndrome and vertebral fractures in up to 78% when doctors look carefully with imaging.[43] What makes this a true hidden thief is that it's frequently missed for years. Patients often chalk up the weight gain, fatigue, and mood changes to stress or aging, while their bones quietly deteriorate. Some people with Cushing's fracture even when their DEXA shows only mild bone loss, because excess cortisol degrades the trabecular honeycomb (Chapter 3) in ways that a standard density measurement can miss. You may be wondering whether the cortisol your body produces during everyday chronic stress can do the same thing. The research suggests it can, though on a smaller scale; studies have linked chronically elevated stress-related cortisol to lower bone density in the spine and increased fracture risk.[44] Luckily, once Cushing's is treated, bone density can improve significantly over the next one to two years. If your osteoporosis doesn't have an obvious explanation, or if you're experiencing unexplained weight gain, easy bruising, or muscle weakness alongside your bone loss, ask your doctor whether screening is appropriate.

Type 2 Diabetes: The Bone Thief That Hides Behind Good Numbers

Type 2 diabetes affects nearly one in three Americans over 65. Unlike the other thieves in this chapter, type 2 diabetes doesn't lower your bone density. People with type 2 diabetes often have normal or even higher-than-average DEXA scores, yet their risk of hip fracture is about 30% higher than in people without diabetes.[45] The culprit is chronically elevated blood sugar, which promotes the buildup of unhealthy substances in bone collagen. Collagen is the flexible scaffolding that gives bones their ability to absorb impact, and that buildup stiffens the scaffolding, making bones more brittle without making them less dense. The result is bones that look strong on a DEXA scan but fracture more easily than the numbers would predict. Standard FRAX also underestimates risk in this group, because it wasn't designed to capture this kind of hidden fragility.[46] The newer FRAXplus calculator we discussed in Chapter 4 now includes an adjustment for type 2 diabetes that accounts for how long you've had the condition, which can give a more accurate picture of your true fracture risk. If you have type 2 diabetes, talk with your doctor about whether your risk assessment should reflect your diabetes, and make the exercise and nutrition strategies in Chapters 7 and 8 a priority.

Chronic Kidney Disease: When Your Bones Lose Their Vitamin D Factory

Your kidneys do more than filter waste. They're responsible for converting vitamin D into its active form, the form your intestines need in order to absorb calcium from food. When kidney function falters, so can your bone strength. Chronic kidney disease is common: it affects about 14% of American adults overall and becomes increasingly prevalent after 65.[47] Many people with early-stage kidney disease have no symptoms at all. If your doctor has noted reduced kidney function on routine bloodwork, ask whether your vitamin D levels, calcium, and PTH should be monitored more closely.

THE HIDDEN DIETARY THIEVES: FOODS THAT STEAL CALCIUM FROM BONES

During my research, I learned that what we eat (and drink) matters more than I realized. Some dietary habits quietly undermine bone health in ways that surprised even me as a physician.

Ultra-Processed Foods and Phosphate Additives

Ultra-processed foods, which are foods far from their natural states, with multiple difficult-to-pronounce ingredients and packaged in bags or boxes, are common culprits. These foods often contain phosphate additives that can disrupt the delicate calcium–phosphate balance in your body. These preservatives essentially pull minerals out of your bone to maintain your blood chemistry. I was shocked to discover how many foods contain these additives, from fast food and processed meats to baked goods and "healthy" frozen meals.

The research on phosphate additives was eye-opening. Reading ingredient lists became a new habit, and I found myself looking for words like "phosphate," "phosphoric acid," or anything containing "phos." Interestingly, naturally occurring organic phosphorus in foods like meat, beans, dairy, and nuts is absorbed much more slowly by the body and doesn't disrupt calcium balance.

My Diet Cola Wake-Up Call

My daily diet cola habit was particularly problematic. Cola drinks combine phosphoric acid with caffeine, both of which are substances that can accelerate bone loss. This was a difficult realization, since I'd been a diet cola drinker for years. Giving up my afternoon diet cola became one of the first concrete changes I made. My dentist congratulated me, too, as cola is terrible for your teeth.

Coffee: The Caffeine Connection

I also cut back on my coffee consumption, from six cups daily down to three. Caffeine increases the amount of calcium lost through your urine. The amount is very small, but for those who drink coffee excessively and skimp on calcium, it adds up. Thankfully, cutting caffeine out entirely isn't necessary for bone health. I'm not sure I could do that! It's also worth noting that it's the caffeine itself, not something unique to coffee, that drives this effect; so, the same applies to energy drinks and heavily caffeinated teas.

The Vitamin D Deficiency Problem

Vitamin D deficiency emerged as another hidden thief I hadn't fully appreciated. As a physician, I knew vitamin D was important for bone health, but I hadn't really considered how dramatically low levels contribute to osteoporosis risk or how common deficiency is.

Remember from Chapter 3 how vitamin D helps you absorb calcium? If you're not getting enough vitamin D, your body will be able to absorb only a small percentage of the calcium in your diet. This means you could be eating plenty of calcium-rich foods and taking calcium supplements, but if your vitamin D is low, most of that calcium will be passing right through your system without ever reaching your bones.

Looking at my own history, I realized I had multiple risk factors for vitamin D deficiency: working indoors all day, diligent sunscreen use, and living in the upper Midwest of the United States, where winter sunlight is too weak to generate adequate vitamin D. After my fractures, my doctor checked my vitamin D level, and I wasn't surprised to find it was low: not severely deficient, but well below optimal.

I live in a northern climate, and I wear sunscreen religiously all summer. All the "healthy" choices that protected my skin were contributing to vitamin D deficiency that weakened my bones. Sometimes, being health-conscious in one area blinds you to risks in another.

I'll discuss the complete vitamin D story, including testing, optimal levels, and supplementation strategies, in detail in Chapter 8.

Did You Know? More than one-third of American adults may have insufficient vitamin D levels. Without adequate vitamin D, your intestines can absorb only 10–15% of the calcium from your food, compared to 30–40% with sufficient levels.[48]

WHEN THIEVES WORK TOGETHER: THE SYNERGISTIC EFFECT

What really concerned me during my research was learning how these factors can work together. A person who's taking corticosteroids who also drinks nothing but coffee and soft drinks, gets poor sleep, and has been through early menopause (or androgen deprivation treatment for prostate cancer) might experience bone loss far exceeding what any single factor would cause alone.

Looking back at my own history, I could see the perfect storm building: early menopause, chronic stress (which elevates bone-damaging cortisol), six cups of coffee a day, taking an SSRI antidepressant for years, and then rapid weight loss without exercising to keep my muscle mass. No wonder my bones were struggling. My osteoporosis likely wasn't due to just one or two specific things, but all together these factors put my bones at risk.

TAKING STOCK OF MY HABITS AND MAKING SUSTAINABLE CHANGES

The encouraging news is that identifying these hidden factors empowers you to act. I started by making a brutally honest inventory of my lifestyle and medical history. How much caffeine was I really consuming? What medications had I taken over the years? How was my sleep quality?

Rather than trying to address everything at once (a recipe for failure in my experience), I tackled one thief at a time. First, I swapped diet cola for ice water with lemon or a splash of orange juice. Next came a review of all of my supplements and medications to ensure I wasn't inadvertently harming my bones. After carefully weighing the risks and benefits, I spoke with my doctor and we decreased, but didn't eliminate, the dosage of the SSRI I'd been taking for decades. The evidence on antidepressants and bone health is still evolving and I am hedging my bet to keep supporting my mental health. Finally, I worked on my stress levels and slowly cut back on the coffee.

The goal is progress and awareness, not perfection. Sometimes, simply recognizing a hidden thief allows you to make small adjustments that meaningfully impact your bone health over time, especially if you do this early in your life.

Understanding all these hidden threats felt overwhelming initially, but it also gave me hope. While I couldn't change my age, genetics, or past medical history, there were powerful interventions that could help rebuild my bone strength, some of which didn't even require a prescription. Armed with the knowledge of what had gone wrong and the emotional resilience I'd been building since my diagnosis, I was finally ready to take action. It was time to fight back against osteoporosis with every tool available, starting with one of the most powerful: exercise.

KEY TAKEAWAYS

- Hidden bone thieves include inflammatory diseases, medications (especially corticosteroids), rapid weight loss, excessive caffeine and alcohol, and chronic stress.
- Early menopause or surgical menopause significantly accelerates bone loss; some women can lose up to 20% of their bone density in the five to seven years following menopause.
- Tackle one bone thief at a time rather than trying to address everything at once; progress matters more than perfection.

PART 2

TREATMENT AND ACTIVE MANAGEMENT

CHAPTER 7

MOVING FOR STRONGER BONES

Exercise That Protects and Builds

When you have osteoporosis, exercise isn't just about general fitness; it becomes actual medicine for your bones. The mechanical stress that physical activity creates sends powerful signals to bone cells (remember those osteoblasts from Chapter 3?), encouraging them to build and strengthen.

Before my diagnosis, my approach to exercise was pretty casual. I walked the dog (when Finnegan wasn't dragging me across lawns), occasionally attended a yoga class, and called it good. After my diagnosis, that lackadaisical attitude was no longer an option. My bones needed intentional, consistent loading to rebuild their strength, and I needed to learn how to provide it safely.

In this chapter, I'll walk you through what the research says about exercise and bone health, including the specific types of exercises that have been shown to protect and build bone strength.

Then I'll share how I applied those principles during my own recovery, including what worked and how I found a sustainable routine after my compression fractures.

YOUR BONES LOVE TO BE CHALLENGED

Your skeleton is remarkably smart. It responds to the forces you place on it by becoming stronger in exactly the areas where strength is needed. Weight-bearing exercises like walking, jogging, dancing, and hiking send "pounding" signals through your bones that tell your bone-building cells, those osteoblasts we talked about, "Hey, we need more reinforcement here!"

The impact doesn't need to be extreme to start sending signals to your bones; even moderate loading tells your osteoblasts to get busy. Think of it this way: if you never challenged your bones, they'd assume they didn't need to be very strong and would gradually weaken. But regular, appropriate stress signals them to maintain and even build strength.

Resistance training provides a different but equally important stimulus. When muscles contract forcefully against resistance, they pull on the bones they're attached to. This tugging encourages those bones to thicken and strengthen at the attachment points. This is why people who lift weights typically have denser bones than those who only do cardio.

Balance and posture work address fall prevention, which is just as important as bone strengthening when you're trying to avoid fractures. Strong postural muscles help combat the forward spine curvature that can develop with vertebral fractures, while good balance reduces your likelihood of taking a dangerous tumble.

BEST EXERCISES

The most important types of exercise are weight-bearing activities (being on your feet; for example, jogging rather than swimming) and resistance training (making your muscles move against a load, like a weight, a resistance band, or even your own body weight).

Check with your doctor before starting a new exercise program, especially if you've already had fractures or haven't exercised in years. If you're already a regular exerciser, great! Make sure you include some exercises specifically for your bones.

EVIDENCE-BASED EXERCISE PRESCRIPTIONS FOR BONE HEALTH

With those principles in mind, let's look at what the research says about the most effective exercises for building and maintaining bone strength. People at different fitness levels need different approaches to maximize the bone-building benefits, so I've organized these recommendations by experience level.

Important: Before You Begin

If you're over 50, haven't exercised regularly, or have any chronic health conditions, discuss these exercises with your healthcare provider before starting. This is especially important if you've had recent fractures, have severe osteoporosis (T-score below –3.0), or experience pain with movement. Ideally, people with recent fractures or severe osteoporosis should develop their exercise program together with a physical therapist who understands bone health.

I realize that not everyone has access to a physical therapist or a personal trainer, whether that's because of cost or simply where you live. If that's your situation, use this chapter as a starting guide, and also seek out books and videos focused on safe, effective exercise for people with osteoporosis. The Bone Health & Osteoporosis Foundation website (bonehealthandosteoporosis.org) offers free resources, and many physical therapists now post instructional content online. The extra effort to find good guidance is worth it. You want to stay safe while exercising and be sure that your routine is actually doing what you need it to do: building bone mass.

Osteoporosis affects a broad group of people with different fitness levels and safety risks. As you read these recommendations, please use common sense. Hiking an uneven trail or working with heavy free weights may be great for a younger person trying to reverse osteopenia, but it would be dangerous for someone older with severe osteoporosis or anyone with recent fractures.

The recommendations below are evidence-based goals to work toward gradually. Start with lighter weights and fewer repetitions than suggested, focusing on perfect form. Fewer repetitions with good form are always better than lots of repetitions with poor form. As you build strength and confidence, you can progressively increase the intensity.

TOP FIVE RESISTANCE EXERCISES FOR BEGINNERS

These exercises require minimal equipment and are appropriate for people newly diagnosed with osteopenia or osteoporosis who have received medical clearance to exercise.

1. CHAIR SQUATS
(Targets: Hips, Thighs, Lower Spine)

How to perform: Stand in front of a sturdy chair with your feet shoulder-width apart. Slowly lower yourself as if sitting down, lightly touching the chair seat, then stand back up without using your hands if possible. Keep your chest up and your knees tracking over your toes.

Goal: 2–3 sets of 10–15 repetitions, 2–3 times per week.

Why it works: Squats load the hip and spine, the two most critical fracture sites, while also building the leg strength needed for daily activities and fall prevention.

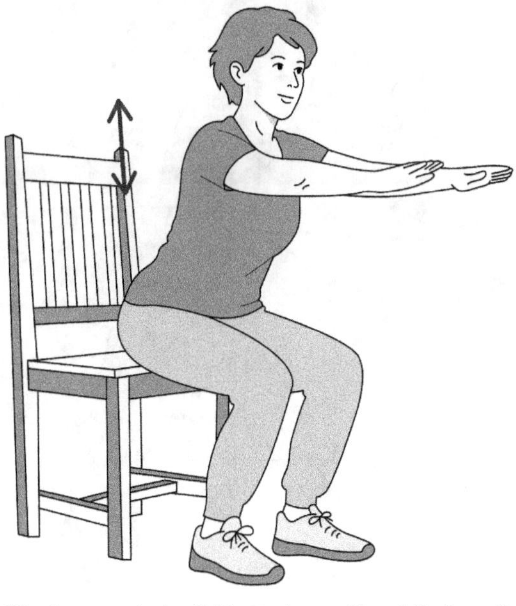

Figure 7.1: Chair squats build leg strength while loading the hip and spine.

2. WALL PUSH-UPS
(Targets: Wrists, Arms, Upper Spine)

How to perform: Stand arm's length from a wall, hands flat against it at shoulder height. Lean toward the wall, bending your elbows, then push back to the starting position. Keep your body in a straight line.

Goal: 2–3 sets of 10–15 repetitions, 2–3 times per week.

Why it works: This exercise safely loads the wrists (an early fracture site) and the bones of the upper body while building functional upper body strength.

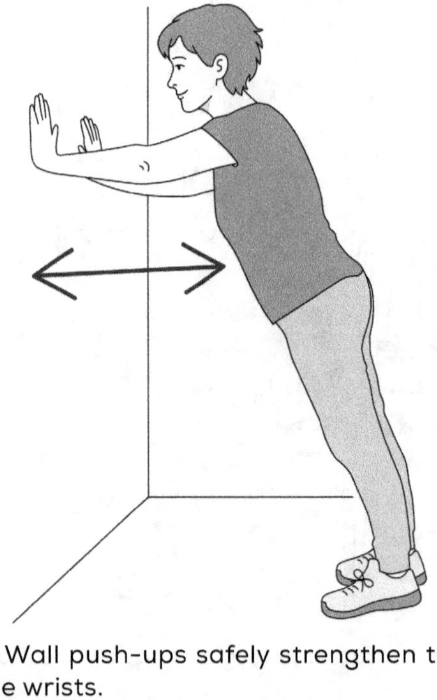

Figure 7.2: Wall push-ups safely strengthen the upper body and load the wrists.

3. STANDING HEEL RAISES
(Targets: Lower Legs, Hips, Spine)

How to perform: Stand near a wall or a counter for light balance support. Rise up onto your toes, hold for 2 seconds, then lower down with control to a gentle but firm landing. The controlled lowering creates beneficial impact.

Goal: 2–3 sets of 15–20 repetitions, 2–3 times per week.

Why it works: The impact of landing stimulates bone formation throughout the lower body and spine. This exercise is easily modifiable: you can increase the impact by coming down more firmly as you get stronger.

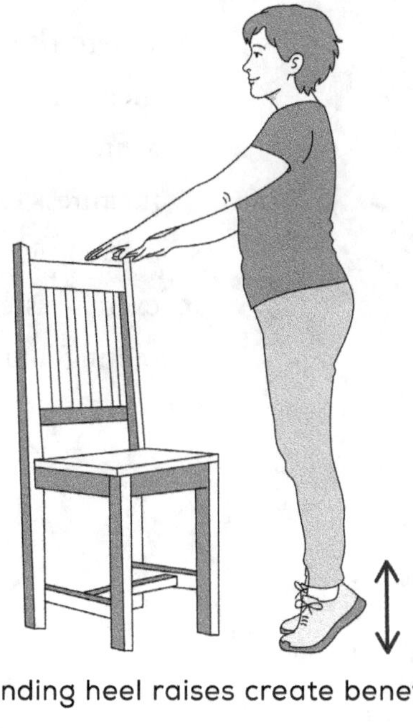

Figure 7.3: Standing heel raises create beneficial impact for the lower body.

4. DUMBBELL OR RESISTANCE BAND ROWS
(Targets: Upper and Mid-Back, Arms)

How to perform: Using light dumbbells (3–5 lbs. to start) or a resistance band, hinge forward slightly at the hips with a straight back. Pull the weights or band toward your ribs, squeezing your shoulder blades together, then slowly lower them again. You can do this standing or with one knee on a bench for support.

Goal: 2–3 sets of 10–12 repetitions, 2–3 times per week.

Why it works: Strengthening the back muscles helps maintain good posture and counteracts the forward curve that can develop with vertebral fractures. The pulling motion loads the arm bones and spine.

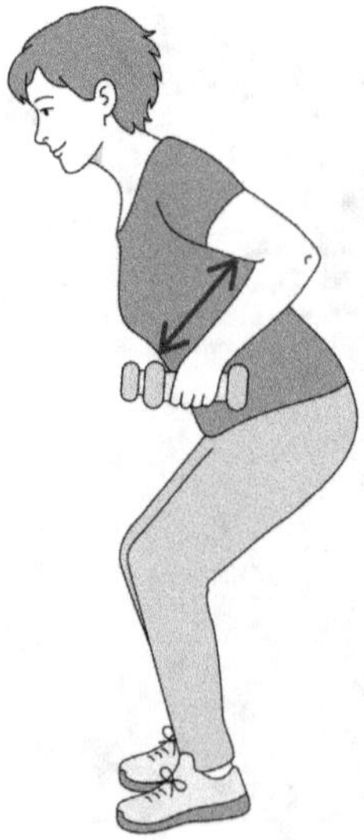

Figure 7.4: Dumbbell rows strengthen the back and improve posture.

When this is not recommended: Avoid if you have acute vertebral compression fractures. Once healed and cleared by your doctor, this exercise is excellent for preventing future fractures.

5. STANDING HIP ABDUCTION
(Targets: Hips, Pelvis)

How to perform: Stand next to a wall or a counter for support. Keeping your leg straight and your toes pointing forward, lift one leg out to the side about 12 inches, hold briefly, then slowly lower. Keep your body upright; don't lean.

Goal: 2–3 sets of 12–15 repetitions per leg, 2–3 times per week. You can add ankle weights (1–2 lbs.) as you progress.

Why it works: This directly targets the hip, the most critical fracture site for maintaining independence. Strong hip abductors also improve balance and reduce fall risk.

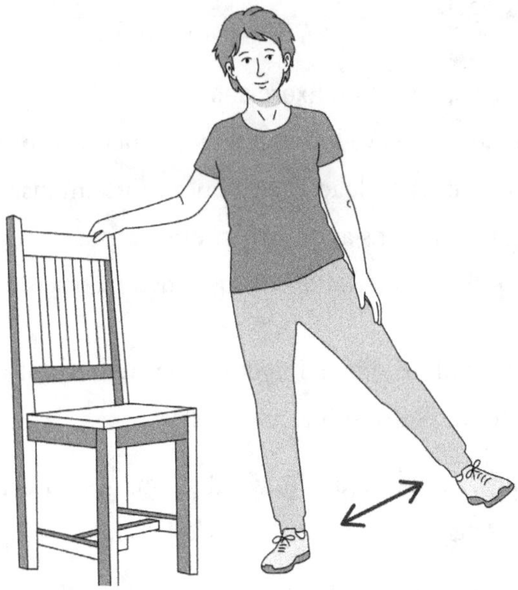

Figure 7.5: Standing hip abduction targets the hip and improves balance.

TOP FIVE RESISTANCE EXERCISES FOR EXPERIENCED EXERCISERS: TRADITIONAL AND EVIDENCE-BASED APPROACHES

If you were already athletic or fit before your diagnosis and have been exercising regularly, your body may be ready for more challenging approaches. The exercises in this section require excellent form, appropriate supervision, and a gradual progression to heavier weights.

Before we begin, let me be clear about something important: walking and light weights are valuable for maintaining bone and overall health. But if your goal is to build significant bone density, the research shows you need more intensity. Remember, your bones adapt to the demands you place on them. If you only ever ask them to support light loads, they have no reason to get stronger.

Traditional Heavy Lifting Exercises

These exercises have long been recommended for experienced exercisers looking to load their bones more intensively. I'm not including illustrations and instructions here, as you should learn how to do these exercises from a qualified instructor.

- Modified deadlifts: Target the entire back of the body, including hips, spine, and legs.
- Bulgarian split squats or weighted lunges: Target the hips and thighs, and improve single-leg stability.
- Overhead press: Loads the shoulders, upper spine, and arms.

- Weighted step-ups: Combine weight-bearing impact with resistance for hips and legs.
- Weighted back extensions: Directly strengthen the muscles supporting the spine.

These exercises are effective, but they require excellent form. Work with a qualified trainer or physical therapist who can ensure you're performing them safely and advancing at the right pace.

Important safety note: Avoid these exercises entirely if you have vertebral fractures or are in the acute phase of recovery from any fracture. Start with the gentler exercises earlier in this chapter and work with your healthcare team before progressing.

The HiRIT Protocol: A Drug-Free Option for Serious Bone-Building

If you're already fit and looking for something more intensive, there's exciting research worth knowing about. High-intensity resistance and impact training (HiRIT) is a supervised exercise protocol that combines heavy weights (80–85% of your maximum capacity) with impact exercises like jumping movements and controlled landings. This combination provides the powerful, novel stimulus that bones need to trigger real rebuilding.

A landmark trial studied postmenopausal women with osteoporosis and osteopenia who followed this program twice weekly for eight months. Participants gained about 3% in lumbar (lower) spine bone density, while the control group lost bone. To put that in perspective, those improvements are comparable to what some medications achieve. Participants also saw a 25–35% increase in muscle strength, better balance, and improved posture. Despite the intensity, the program had an excellent safety record, with no fractures during the trial.[49]

I'll be honest: when I first learned about HiRIT, I was skeptical. Like many doctors, I'd been taught that people with osteoporosis should avoid heavy weights and impact. But this research changed my thinking. For people who are determined and disciplined enough to pursue it with proper supervision, HiRIT offers a non-pharmaceutical path to meaningful improvement in bone density, strength, and balance: the very factors that protect against fractures.

There are important caveats. HiRIT should only be done under close, ongoing supervision by professionals trained in this specific protocol. This is not a program to attempt on your own or with a general fitness trainer. It requires precise form, appropriate weight progression, and constant monitoring to be both safe and effective. It also won't be right for everyone. You need medical clearance and access to qualified supervision, which isn't available everywhere (look for exercise professionals with BoneFit certification through the Bone Health and Osteoporosis Foundation). But if you're someone who thrives on challenging workouts and wants to take an active role in strengthening your bones, it's worth investigating.

The Bottom Line for Highly Motivated Exercisers

Whether you choose traditional heavy resistance exercises or pursue a formal HiRIT program, the evidence is clear. Your bones can handle more than you might think, and they need that challenge to get stronger. Work with qualified professionals, progress gradually, and give your body the powerful stimulus it needs to rebuild.

WEIGHT-BEARING CARDIOVASCULAR EXERCISE

While resistance training provides the most potent bone-building stimulus, weight-bearing cardio activities add valuable variety and additional benefits for bone health, cardiovascular fitness, and overall well-being.

Weight-bearing activities require your bones and muscles to work against gravity while supporting your body weight. The impact and loading patterns stimulate bone formation throughout your skeleton. If you've had a recent fracture, check with your doctor or physical therapist before any high-impact exercise.

Effective weight-bearing cardio options include:

- **Walking:** The most accessible option, and sometimes the only option if you have recent fractures or very severe osteoporosis. Aim for 30–60 minutes most days of the week. While walking alone provides modest bone benefits, it improves cardiovascular health and reduces fall risk through improved balance and leg strength. Walking on varied terrain (hills, trails) or at a brisker pace increases the bone-building benefit.

- **Jogging/running:** Provides greater impact than walking. If you were a runner before your diagnosis and have medical clearance, you can continue with appropriate precautions. Start conservatively, with 15–20 minutes two to three times weekly, and increase gradually.

- **Jumping exercises:** Provide high-impact loading that can be particularly effective for bone building. Research shows that even brief daily jumping sessions (10–20 jumps) can significantly improve bone density in healthy individuals. Options include jump rope, jumping jacks, or simply skipping or hopping in place. Start with small jumps, and progress gradually.[50]

Did You Know? When it comes to jumping for bone health, more isn't necessarily better. Research shows bone cells respond strongly to the first 10–40 jumps, then become temporarily "deaf" to further impact. That's why brief sessions with rests between jumps work better than marathon jumping workouts.[51]

- **Dancing:** Combines impact, weight-bearing, and varied movement patterns that challenge balance and coordination. Whether it's Zumba or just dancing to your favorite music at home, this counts as bone-healthy exercise while being enjoyable and social.
- **Hiking:** Offers the benefits of walking plus the added challenge of uneven terrain and elevation changes, which enhance both bone loading and balance training. Start on well-maintained trails, and progress to more challenging terrain as your confidence builds.
- **Stair climbing:** This activity provides excellent loading to the hips and spine. It's better to use actual stairs rather than a stair-climbing machine, as the impact on

the skeleton is a bit greater. Start with just a few flights, and build gradually.

- **Tennis, pickleball, or similar racquet sports:** These provide impact, varied movement patterns, and social engagement. The stop-and-start nature and lateral movements offer diverse bone-loading patterns.

Activities to Avoid or Modify

Swimming and cycling, while excellent for cardiovascular fitness, are not weight-bearing and provide minimal bone-building benefits. They're fine to include for overall fitness, but they shouldn't replace weight-bearing activities in your bone health program.

How Much Weight-Bearing Cardio?

Aim for 30–60 minutes of weight-bearing activity on most days of the week, in addition to your resistance training sessions. This can be broken into shorter segments; three 10-minute walks provide similar benefits to one 30-minute walk. The key is consistency.

BALANCE EXERCISES: YOUR BEST DEFENSE AGAINST FALLS

For anyone with osteoporosis, preventing falls is just as important as building stronger bones. After all, the most dangerous fractures (hip and spine) almost always result from a fall. The good news is that balance is not a fixed trait; it's a skill that improves with practice at any age. Research shows that balance training can reduce falls in older adults by up to 40%, with the greatest benefit coming from regular, progressive practice.

Balance depends on the coordination of multiple body systems: your vision, inner ear, joint sensors, and muscle strength all work together to keep you upright. As we age, each of these systems can decline gradually, often without our noticing, until a stumble or near-fall sounds the alarm. Illness, inactivity, and certain medications can accelerate the decline. But targeted balance exercises can retrain these systems and restore confidence in your steadiness. The American Physical Therapy Association recommends balance training at least two to three days per week, emphasizing that exercises should be progressively challenging; a slight wobble means your body is learning.

Getting Started: Exercises Anyone Can Do

Start near a kitchen counter, sturdy chair back, or wall so you can catch yourself if needed. Having a friend or partner nearby is also a good idea. Begin with two-hand support, progress to one hand, and eventually try hands-free. Don't rush the progression. Move to the next level only when you can hold steady for at least 10 seconds at the current one:

- **Single-leg stand:** Lift one foot slightly off the ground and hold for up to 30 seconds, then switch legs. Aim for three to five repetitions on each side. This is one of the most effective and well-studied balance exercises, and you can easily, and quietly, work it into daily life. Practice while waiting for the coffee to brew or talking on the phone.
- **Heel-to-toe standing and walking:** Place one foot directly in front of the other so the heel of the front foot touches

the toes of the back foot. Hold this tandem stance for up to 30 seconds. When that feels manageable, try walking forward in this heel-to-toe pattern, as if on a tightrope, for 10–15 steps. Then try walking backward in the same way.

- **Weight shifts:** Stand with feet hip-width apart. Shift your weight slowly onto one foot, lifting the other slightly off the floor. Hold for a few seconds, return to center, and repeat on the other side. This trains your body to recover from the small weight transfers that happen naturally during walking.

Stepping It Up: More Challenging Balance Work

Once the basic exercises feel routine, it's time to add complexity. Harder balance challenges force your body to adapt in ways that better prepare you for real-world situations, such as uneven sidewalks, icy parking lots, or a pet unexpectedly underfoot:

- **Sidestepping:** Facing a counter for safety, step sideways in one direction with your toes pointed straight ahead, then return the other way. This strengthens the hip muscles that stabilize you during everyday lateral movements, like stepping around furniture or catching your balance when jostled. For an extra challenge, loop a resistance band around your ankles.

- **Clock stepping:** Imagine a clock face on the floor around you. Have a partner call out positions, such as "12 o'clock," "3 o'clock," "9 o'clock," and "6 o'clock"; quickly step to each position before returning to center. This trains reaction time alongside balance, which matters because real-world slips and trips happen fast.

- **Tai chi:** This ancient practice is one of the most thoroughly researched balance improvers, with studies showing significant reductions in fall rates among older adults. Its slow, flowing movements develop balance, leg strength, and body awareness simultaneously. Many community centers and senior programs offer classes specifically designed for fall prevention. If a class isn't available near you, guided video programs can be a good starting point.

Once you're comfortable with any balance exercise, increase the difficulty by reducing support (two hands to one hand to none), adding movement (arm reaches, head turns), narrowing your stance, or standing on a less stable surface like a folded towel or a pillow. Closing your eyes during familiar exercises removes visual input and forces your body to rely more on muscle and joint feedback. Only try this near a support surface and when you feel confident with your eyes open.

The beauty of balance training is that it requires no equipment and very little time. Even 5–10 minutes a day, woven into activities you're already doing, can make a real difference. If your balance feels particularly unsteady or if you've had a recent fall, consider working with a physical therapist who can assess your specific risk factors and design a program tailored to your needs. Some physical therapists specialize in balance and fall prevention, and a personalized program can be the safest way to start.

Putting It All Together

A comprehensive bone-building exercise program includes resistance training, weight-bearing cardio, and balance and flexibility work:

- **Resistance training:** Two to three sessions per week, allowing at least one day of rest between sessions for the same muscle groups
- **Weight-bearing cardio:** Most days of the week, 30–60 minutes total (can be accumulated throughout the day)
- **Balance and flexibility work:** Daily or several times weekly (single-leg stands, heel-to-toe walking, gentle stretching)

Beginners might do a wide range of resistance exercises each session, or, if that feels overwhelming, alternate between upper body exercises one day and lower body exercises the next. Advanced exercisers who already have established workout routines should ensure these bone-specific exercises are part of their program, even if they're doing other exercises as well.

An important aspect of exercising is consistency. Doing moderate exercise regularly will build stronger bones than sporadic intense workouts. Start where you are, progress gradually, and remember that every session is an investment in your future strength and independence.

MY EXERCISE JOURNEY: PUTTING THE EVIDENCE INTO PRACTICE

Reading about evidence-based exercise is one thing. Figuring out how to actually do it after compression fractures, when you're scared of reinjury and uncertain what your body can handle, is something else entirely. Here's how I navigated that gap.

Learning What My Body Could Handle

After my compression fractures, I had to completely relearn what exercise meant for my body. Working with a physical therapist was invaluable, because I needed to understand which movements would help my bones without risking additional injury.

Some exercises that seemed obviously beneficial turned out to be problematic. Traditional sit-ups and crunches, for example, involve forward spine flexion under load. That's exactly the movement pattern that can compress vulnerable vertebrae. I had to learn new ways to strengthen my core without putting my healing spine at risk.

Forward bending with weight became another no-go. This meant modifying how I picked things up, how I gardened, and even how I loaded the dishwasher. It felt restrictive initially, but learning proper body mechanics became second nature with practice.

Building Strength Safely

My physical therapist and I started with many of the beginner exercises described earlier in this chapter, adapting them to my recovery stage. Heel drops became one of my favorites because they're simple but effective. Standing next to a chair for balance, I'd rise on my toes, hold for two seconds, then slowly lower down to a gentle thud. Completely controllable in terms of intensity, but still providing real impact stimulus for my bones.

Wall push-ups, another staple from the beginner list, replaced floor push-ups during my early recovery. As I got stronger, I progressed to inclined push-ups against stairs, then eventually to knee push-ups.

Chair-assisted squats helped me rebuild hip and thigh strength. I'd sit in the chair, then stand up without using my hands if possible, and slowly lower down until I was just touching the seat. This movement pattern is important for daily activities and provides excellent bone loading.

Back extension exercises became essential for strengthening the muscles supporting my spine, though I had to learn the safe way to do them. Instead of lying face-down and arching backward, I learned to do them standing with my hands on my hips, gently arching backward while engaging my back muscles.

Rediscovering Balance

My balance had suffered more than I realized, probably due to all the time I'd spent lying on the couch healing. Simple activities like standing on one foot or walking heel-to-toe suddenly felt challenging and a little scary, honestly. But working on my balance proved both rewarding and important for fall prevention.

Single-leg stands became a daily practice. Holding onto a chair for light support, I'd lift one foot slightly off the ground and try to hold it for 10–30 seconds. As my confidence returned, I could let go of the chair for brief periods.

Heel-to-toe walking sounds simple, but it requires surprising concentration and stability. Walking in a straight line, placing my heel directly in front of the toes of the other foot with each step, challenged my balance in ways that translated to better stability in daily life.

> **Did You Know?** Exercise programs that challenge balance can reduce falls in older adults by up to 40%, with the greatest benefit from higher doses of balance-specific training. Since almost all hip and wrist fractures result from falls, preventing falls may be just as important as building bone density.[52,53]

The Mental Transformation

The biggest change wasn't physical but mental. Exercise transformed from something I did when I felt like it to something I needed for my health, like taking blood pressure medication. The diagnosis eliminated the luxury of making excuses about being too busy or too tired.

The shift didn't happen overnight. Some days, I still struggled with motivation, especially during the early months when movement was uncomfortable and my confidence was shaky. But gradually, exercise became less about forcing myself to do something I should do and more about actively investing in my future independence.

I learned to celebrate small victories. Moving up from the 10-pound weights to the 12-pound ones. Carrying groceries without thinking twice. These weren't dramatic fitness transformations, but they represented genuine progress that accumulated over time.

Making It Sustainable

Research clearly shows that sporadic exercise provides minimal benefit for bone health. Consistency matters even more than intensity. A hard workout once a month, even if it loads your skeleton well, is not an effective strategy. So, I had to find ways to make movement sustainable and enjoyable rather than punitive.

I mixed different types of activities throughout the week to prevent boredom and ensure I addressed weight-bearing, resistance, balance, and posture work. Some days focused on strength, others on balance, and some combined multiple elements. I no longer held the leash, but I joined my husband on the nightly dog-walks.

Working with healthcare providers who understood osteoporosis made a huge difference. They helped me distinguish between the normal discomfort of challenging muscles and warning signs of potential injury. The goal became progressive overload (gradually increasing the challenge over time) rather than dramatic immediate changes.

Finding My New Normal

About eight months into my exercise journey, I realized that movement had become a source of confidence rather than anxiety. Each completed workout proved to me that I was getting stronger, not weaker. Each balance exercise successfully completed reminded me that I was taking control of my fall risk.

The woman who had once treated exercise as optional had

become someone who prioritized it as essential medicine. Not only because I had to, but because I could feel the difference it was making in my strength and balance. I found myself feeling more capable in my day-to-day life.

As I planned my exercise routine and felt hopeful about rebuilding my bone strength, I knew that movement was only part of the equation. My skeleton needed quality building materials for the construction project ahead, and that meant taking a hard look at how I'd been fueling my bones for all these years.

KEY TAKEAWAYS

- Weight-bearing exercise and resistance training are both essential medicine for bones; they signal your skeleton to build and maintain strength.
- Balance and posture exercises are equally important, because preventing falls is just as critical as building bone strength.
- Start slowly and progress gradually, especially if you have fractures or severe osteoporosis. Working with a physical therapist can ensure you're exercising safely, but books, videos, and online resources can guide you if professional help isn't accessible.

CHAPTER 8

NUTRITION AND BONE HEALTH

Calcium, Vitamin D, and Building a Bone-Friendly Diet

During those months of careful movement and gradual recovery, I realized that exercise alone couldn't rebuild my bone strength. My skeleton needed quality raw materials for the construction project ahead, and that meant honestly examining how I'd been feeding my bones for decades.

This wasn't just about taking calcium supplements, though that became part of it. I discovered that bone health depends on a complex interplay of nutrients, and some of my daily food choices had been working against my skeleton for years without my realizing it.

BEYOND THE CALCIUM BASICS

Everyone knows bones need calcium, but I learned that getting calcium into your bones is more complicated than just swallowing pills. It's also confusing, as, unlike with vitamin D, testing your blood calcium levels isn't an accurate way to tell whether you're getting enough calcium in your diet. As we saw in Chapter 3, your body controls the level of calcium in your blood very tightly; it works hard to keep it in the "normal" range so your heart can function properly. This means you can have a normal blood calcium level because your body is dipping into your bone bank every day to achieve that, while still having a calcium-deficient diet or not absorbing enough of the calcium you do eat.

Whole, healthy foods are better than supplements, but I realized I wasn't getting enough calcium from my diet. Calcium supplements are available in calcium carbonate and calcium citrate forms. While they both provide calcium, they are slightly different. Calcium citrate emerged as my preferred supplement form because it absorbs well even without stomach acid and proved gentler on my digestion than calcium carbonate. But timing and absorption turned out to matter as much as the total amount.

Your body can only absorb about 500 mg of calcium at once, so I had to split my intake. I aimed for 1,200 mg daily from food and supplements combined, spreading my intake throughout the day. Taking calcium with my morning coffee turned out to be counterproductive; caffeine can increase calcium excretion, possibly canceling out some of the benefit.

OTHER NUTRIENTS FOR BONE HEALTH

Vitamin D3 was equally important, since it's essential for calcium absorption and increases the toughness of bones. I started taking it with meals containing some fat to optimize absorption.

While the Institute of Medicine recommends 600–800 IU daily for most adults, you'll need more if you have vitamin D deficiency. If you have osteoporosis, you should be monitoring your vitamin D levels. This means asking your healthcare provider to periodically order a simple blood test. Too much can cause abnormally high calcium levels in the blood, calcium deposits in the arteries, and kidney damage. More isn't always better![54] We'll discuss more about this later.

Vitamin K2 for bone health was completely new to me, but research shows that it helps to direct calcium into bones and away from arteries, where it can cause problems. This was particularly relevant since I had some cardiovascular risk factors. I started taking 100 mcg daily, in the MK-7 form that helps direct calcium into the bones rather than into the arteries. Vitamin K can interfere with blood thinners like warfarin, so talk to your doctor before using it if you take that type of medicine.

Magnesium is needed for bone health. It helps your body use vitamin D properly and supports the hormones that control bone building and bone breakdown. Too much magnesium can cause diarrhea, and those with kidney problems should ask their doctor before supplementing. Between 200 and 400 mg of magnesium is recommended daily, between food sources and supplements.

Collagen peptides have been shown in some recent studies to improve bone density. Specifically, 5 g (5,000 mg) of Type I collagen peptides (the type of collagen bones are made of) has been shown to be effective when combined with adequate calcium and vitamin D.[55] Interestingly, the collagen gets broken down into fragments in your digestive system. When your bones notice lots of nice bone-building materials in the bloodstream, they take the hint and start building. It comes in a powder you stir into a drink. Hint: While it's flavorless, it mixes better in a hot drink than a cold one. Unfortunately for vegetarians, there's no true natural vegetarian source of collagen. It's an animal product made from bovine (cow) or marine sources.

REAL FOOD MAKES THE DIFFERENCE

While supplements filled gaps, I learned that whole foods should form the foundation of bone-healthy nutrition. I began prioritizing foods that naturally provide bone-supporting nutrients rather than relying primarily on pills.

Greek yogurt became a breakfast staple; one cup provides about 250 mg of calcium plus high-quality protein. I switched to fortified plant milks for smoothies, though I discovered that calcium content varies dramatically between brands. Reading labels became essential. Some brands of plant milk have extraordinarily little calcium, while others have more calcium than dairy milk.

Sardines might not sound appetizing, but they're nutritional powerhouses for bones. One small can provides about 380 mg of calcium plus vitamin D and omega-3 fatty acids. I learned to mash them into pasta sauces or eat them on crackers, which was an acquired taste that became surprisingly enjoyable. Try adding a few sardines to steamed rice with seaweed flakes and wasabi mayo for a Japanese twist.

Leafy greens like collard greens, kale, and bok choy offer calcium in a form that's well-absorbed, unlike spinach, where the calcium gets bound up with oxalates. Bok choy is the mildest high-calcium green and a good one to add to your diet first. I started adding leafy greens to stir-fries and soups rather than relegating them to occasional side dishes.

Almonds became my go-to snack. One ounce provides about 75 mg of calcium plus healthy fats, protein, and vitamin E. I kept pre-portioned bags in my car and office to avoid less nutritious impulse choices.

AVOID BONE-DEPLETING INGREDIENTS: PHOSPHATES AND EXCESSIVE CAFFEINE

In Chapter 6, we saw that ultra-processed foods and their phosphate additives can work against your bone health goals. Reading ingredient lists became second nature, and I learned to recognize and limit the hidden phosphates in packaged foods.

As I mentioned earlier, I had to give up my diet cola habit and reduce my coffee intake. Both changes proved surprisingly difficult but necessary for my bone health.

THE VITAMIN D EQUATION: SUNLIGHT, FOOD, AND SUPPLEMENTS

Understanding vitamin D became important in my bone health journey, because no matter how much calcium you consume, it won't reach your bones without adequate vitamin D. This vitamin (which is technically a hormone) acts as the gatekeeper for calcium absorption, and getting enough proved more complicated than I'd expected.

Getting Vitamin D from Sunlight

Our bodies are designed to produce vitamin D from sunlight exposure. When UVB rays hit your skin, they trigger a chemical reaction that converts cholesterol into vitamin D3. It's remarkably efficient; just 10–15 minutes of midday sun exposure on your arms and legs can produce about 3,000–5,000 IU of vitamin D in lighter-skinned individuals.

But here's where it gets tricky. The amount of vitamin D your skin produces depends on numerous factors: your latitude (the farther you are from the equator, the weaker the UVB rays), the season (winter sunlight is too weak for vitamin D production in most of the northern hemisphere), time of day (UVB is strongest between 10 a.m. and 3 p.m.), skin pigmentation (darker skin requires more sun exposure), and age (our ability to produce vitamin D decreases as we age). What about sunscreen? Sunscreen use (SPF 30 blocks about 97% of UVB rays), can reduce vitamin D production. In practice, however, most people don't apply sunscreen thickly enough to fully block vitamin D synthesis, and studies haven't found that regular sunscreen use leads to deficiency.

Living in the upper Midwest United States, I realized I was getting virtually no vitamin D from sunlight for about half the year. Even in summer, my mostly indoor lifestyle meant I wasn't producing much. I needed to focus on dietary sources and supplementation.

Food Sources of Vitamin D

Unlike calcium, which is abundant in many foods, vitamin D occurs naturally in very few foods. Fatty fish are the best natural sources; a 3-ounce serving of salmon provides about 570 IU of vitamin D, while the same amount of canned tuna offers about 150 IU. Sardines, which I was already eating for calcium, also provide about 45 IU per can.

Other natural sources are more modest. One large egg yolk contains about 40 IU, and beef liver provides around 50 IU per 3-ounce serving. Mushrooms exposed to UV light can offer significant amounts, with some varieties providing up to 400 IU per serving; however, most commercially grown mushrooms contain very little unless specifically treated.

Given the limited natural food sources, fortified foods (foods with added nutrients like calcium or other vitamins and minerals) became important in my diet. Fortified milk provides about 120 IU of vitamin D per cup, though I often chose fortified almond milk, which offers similar amounts. Orange juice is often fortified with 100 IU per cup. Many breakfast cereals are fortified, though the amounts vary widely by brand.

Looking at these numbers, I realized why vitamin D deficiency is so common. Even with a diet rich in fatty fish, fortified dairy, and eggs, it's difficult to reach the 800–1,000 IU daily recommendation through food alone, especially during winter months when sunlight can't contribute.

Understanding Your Vitamin D Levels

Getting your vitamin D level checked regularly is important. The blood test your doctor orders (called 25-hydroxyvitamin D, sometimes written as 25(OH)D on your lab report) reflects your body's total vitamin D from all sources: sunlight, food, and supplements combined. Insurance often covers this blood test annually when you have a diagnosis of osteoporosis or osteopenia, with testing covered more often if your level is found to be low.

In the United States, results are typically reported in ng/mL (nanograms per milliliter). Here's what those numbers mean:

Vitamin D Level	Status	Guidelines and Clinical Notes
Below 12 ng/mL (30 nmol/L)	Severe deficiency	Supplementation shows the clearest bone health benefits in this range.
12-20 ng/mL (30-50 nmol/L)	Deficient	Supplementation is strongly recommended to reach safe levels.
20-30 ng/mL (50-75 nmol/L)	Insufficient	May benefit from supplementation, especially for protecting bone health.
30-40 ng/mL (75-100 nmol/L)	Adequate	Generally considered adequate for maintaining bone health.
40-50 ng/mL (100-125 nmol/L)	Ideal	Considered the optimal target range for bone strength.
Above 50 ng/mL (125 nmol/L)	Potentially excessive	Provides no additional bone benefit and carries possible risks.

Traditional recommendations suggest targeting levels of at least 30 ng/mL (75 nmol/L) for optimal bone health, with most experts preferring 40-50 ng/mL (100-125 nmol/L).

When and How to Supplement

This is important: vitamin D supplementation provides the clearest bone health benefits for people with documented deficiency. However, multiple recent studies confirm that if your levels are already adequate, taking more vitamin D won't make your bones stronger and might even increase fracture risk in some populations.

This means supplementation should be targeted, not universal. I had my levels checked, confirmed they were low, and then started supplementing. Three months later, I had them rechecked to ensure the dose was adequate; levels typically plateau around this timepoint.

For those who need supplementation, vitamin D3 (sometimes listed on bottles as cholecalciferol) is significantly more effective than vitamin D2 (ergocalciferol). Studies show D3 may be roughly twice as effective at raising and maintaining vitamin D levels, and it stays active in your body for longer, meaning more sustained benefits.[56] When I started supplementing, I specifically looked for vitamin D3 on the label.

Dosing depends on your starting level and individual factors. For people with documented deficiency, doses of 1,000–2,000 IU daily are common. It can also be taken in larger weekly doses by prescription (especially helpful to quickly bring up exceptionally low levels). I take 2,000 IU daily based on my doctor's recommendation and my initial blood levels.

Timing matters for optimal absorption. Vitamin D is fat-soluble, which means it absorbs best when taken with meals containing some fat. I take mine with lunch, which usually includes nuts or avocado. Taking it with a meal also means I'm less likely to forget it compared to other times.

Why We Need Both Calcium and Vitamin D

What really drove home vitamin D's importance was learning about how it worked alongside calcium. The synergy made sense once I understood the mechanisms. As we discussed in Chapter 6, calcium provides the building material, vitamin D ensures that material gets absorbed (increasing absorption from about 10–15% to 30–40%), and together they work to maintain the delicate balance your skeleton needs.

Taking vitamin D by itself doesn't seem to lower the risk of broken bones in healthy adults who aren't low in vitamin D, but studies have found that older adults who take both vitamin D (800–1,000 IU) and calcium (1,000–1,200 mg) each day have modestly reduced fracture risk. The benefit appears strongest in people who have low baseline levels of vitamin D or calcium and in elderly populations.[57,58]

My Vitamin D Strategy

After learning all this, I developed a multipronged approach. I get sensible sun exposure when possible: about 10–15 minutes on my arms and legs most days during the summer. That turned out to be a mood-booster, too! I prioritize vitamin-D-rich foods, including fatty fish twice weekly and fortified milk or almond milk daily. I take a 2,000 IU vitamin D3 supplement with a meal each day. And I have my levels rechecked annually to ensure my approach is working.

Understanding vitamin D's role transformed it from just another supplement I was supposed to take into a crucial partner in my bone health strategy. Knowing my actual levels removed the guesswork and allowed me to supplement intelligently rather than blindly. For anyone with osteoporosis or at risk for it, I can't overemphasize the value of having your vitamin D level tested rather than just assuming supplementation will help.

MAKING PRACTICAL CHANGES: TASTY SUBSTITUTIONS AND MEAL PLANS

Rather than overhauling my entire diet overnight (a strategy I knew would fail), I made gradual substitutions that felt sustainable. I added fortified dairy or almond milk instead of a low-nutrient flavored creamer to my morning coffee. Water with lemon took the place of an afternoon diet cola. Mixed nuts became my desk snack, replacing processed chips or crackers.

I committed to preparing at least one meal daily primarily from whole foods: vegetables, lean protein, whole grains, and healthy fats. This single change improved my nutrient intake substantially while reducing my exposure to problematic additives.

Meal planning became more intentional. Greek yogurt parfaits with berries and nuts for breakfast provided calcium and protein. Salmon salads for lunch delivered omega-3 fatty acids, vitamin D, and high-quality protein. Protein, along with micronutrients such as zinc, magnesium, and B vitamins, also supports bone health. A healthy diet with plenty of fruits, veggies, and lean protein is important. I focused on abundance rather than restriction, adding nutritious options that naturally crowded out less healthy choices.

SUPPLEMENTS AS INSURANCE

Finding the right supplement routine took some experimentation. Calcium citrate worked best taken twice daily with meals, remembering those absorption limits I'd learned about. Vitamin D3 went with my largest meal of the day to optimize absorption. I learned to take vitamin K2 alongside vitamin D since they work synergistically, and both are absorbed better with a fatty meal. Below is the schedule that has worked for me, but not everyone will want to, or be able to, spread things out to three times daily.

The timing became routine:

- 200 mg calcium citrate with breakfast

- 2,000 IU vitamin D3, 100 mcg K2, and 200 mg magnesium glycinate with lunch
- 200 mg calcium citrate and a multivitamin with minerals at supper

If my diet has been stellar on a particular day and full of calcium and protein (like the sample diet at the end of this chapter), I might skip my evening calcium supplement. If my diet hasn't been so stellar, I might up the calcium citrate to 400 mg with supper. Putting the supplement bottles out on the dining table next to the salt and pepper helped me remember to take them with my meals. I worked hard, though, to get my bone-supporting nutrients from food as much as possible.

THE BIGGER PICTURE

One of the most encouraging aspects of eating for bone health was discovering that it supported my overall health at the same time. The same dietary pattern that strengthens bones (emphasizing whole foods, adequate protein, plenty of fruits and vegetables, and minimal processing) also benefits heart health, brain function, and weight management.

This comprehensive approach made the changes feel empowering rather than restrictive. I wasn't just eating for my bones; I was nourishing my entire body in ways that would pay dividends in multiple ways.

Adequate protein became particularly important, since bone is about 50% protein by volume. The collagen matrix that gives bones their flexibility requires a consistent amino acid supply. I aimed for protein at each meal rather than concentrating it all at dinner as I'd done previously.

THE COMPLETE STRONG BONES FOOD LIST

I've shared some of my own food choices and changes throughout this chapter: the Greek yogurt breakfasts, the sardines I learned to enjoy, and almonds as my go-to snack. But I want to provide you with a more comprehensive guide to bone-supporting foods so you can build an eating pattern that works for your preferences and budget.

The foods below are organized by category, with information about their key bone-building nutrients. Remember that whole foods should form the foundation of your bone health nutrition, with supplements filling in the nutritional gaps. While I've included serving sizes and nutrient amounts to help with meal planning, you don't need to obsess over hitting exact numbers at every meal; focus instead on consistently including bone-healthy foods throughout your day and week.

DAIRY AND DAIRY ALTERNATIVES

Dairy products are among the richest and most easily absorbed sources of calcium, and many are also fortified with vitamin D.

Food and Serving Size	Key Nutrients	Additional Notes
Cow's milk (1 cup)	Calcium: 300 mg Protein: 8 g	Often fortified with vitamin D (check labels); budget-friendly option
Greek yogurt (1 cup)	Calcium: 250–300 mg Protein: 15–20 g	Often contains vitamin D; provides probiotics for gut health; choose plain varieties to avoid added sugars
Cheese, hard varieties (e.g., cheddar, Parmesan) (1 oz)	Calcium: 200–250 mg Protein: 7 g	Also provides vitamin K2; a little goes a long way due to concentrated nutrients
Cottage cheese (1 cup)	Calcium: 125–150 mg Protein: 25 g	Lower in calcium than other dairy, but an excellent protein source; budget-friendly
Fortified plant milk (soy, almond, oat) (1 cup)	Calcium: 300–450 mg (when fortified) Vitamin D: often 100–140 IU	Soy milk provides 7–8 g protein, almond/oat milk typically 1–2 g; fortification varies: read labels and shake well before pouring

FISH, MEAT, EGG, AND PLANT PROTEIN

Fish, other animal proteins, and plant-based proteins all contribute to bone health through protein and various minerals. Aim for 0.8 grams per kg of your body weight (0.36 grams per pound of body weight) daily. This will end up being between 45 and 75 grams for most people.

Food and Serving Size	Key Nutrients	Additional Notes
Salmon, wild-caught (3 oz cooked)	Calcium: 180 mg (with bones in canned) Vitamin D: 570 IU Protein: 17 g	One of the best natural sources of vitamin D; also provides omega-3s
Rainbow trout, farmed (3 oz)	Vitamin D: 600 IU Protein: 20 g	One of the highest vitamin D contents among fish; mild flavor
Mackerel, canned (3 oz)	Vitamin D: 450–500 IU Protein: 20 g	Often overlooked, but comparable to salmon for vitamin D; rich flavor
Sardines, canned with bones (3.75 oz can)	Calcium: 350–380 mg Vitamin D: 150–200 IU Protein: 23 g	Budget-friendly; the bones are soft and edible, and they provide most of the calcium
Tuna, canned (3 oz)	Vitamin D: 150 IU Protein: 20 g	Budget-friendly; lower in calcium than sardines but still a good vitamin D source

PROTEIN SOURCES: OTHER ANIMAL PROTEINS

Food and Serving Size	Key Nutrients	Additional Notes
Chicken or turkey (3 oz cooked)	Protein: 25–27 g	Provides zinc and B vitamins that support bone health; versatile and budget-friendly
Eggs (1 large)	Vitamin D: 40 IU (in yolk) Protein: 6 g	Also provides vitamin K2; budget-friendly; the vitamin D is in the yolk, not the white
Lean beef (3 oz cooked)	Protein: 25 g	Provides zinc and vitamin K2; choose grass-fed when possible for higher omega-3 content
Pork tenderloin or loin (3 oz cooked)	Protein: 22–24 g	Provides thiamin (vitamin B1) and zinc; choose lean cuts to minimize saturated fat

PROTEIN SOURCES: PLANT-BASED

Food and Serving Size	Key Nutrients	Additional Notes
Tofu, calcium-set (½ cup)	Calcium: 250–750 mg Protein: 10 g	Only calcium-set tofu provides significant calcium; check ingredients for "calcium sulfate" or "calcium chloride"
Tempeh (½ cup)	Calcium: 90 mg Protein: 15 g	Provides probiotics and is less processed than many meat alternatives
Edamame (1 cup)	Calcium: 100 mg Protein: 17 g	Also provides magnesium and other minerals
Lentils and beans (1 cup cooked)	Calcium: 40–80 mg Protein: 15–18 g	Also provide magnesium, zinc, and other trace minerals; budget-friendly; legumes provide multiple bone-supporting nutrients

VEGETABLES AND LEAFY GREENS: BEST CHOICES (LOW OXALATE, HIGH CALCIUM ABSORPTION)

Dark leafy greens can be excellent calcium sources, but absorption varies significantly depending on their oxalate content. (Oxalate is a natural compound found in some vegetables.)

Food and Serving Size	Key Nutrients	Additional Notes
Collard greens, cooked (1 cup)	Calcium: 270 mg Vitamin K: 770 mcg	Excellent absorption (about 50% vs. 30% from dairy); also provides magnesium; budget-friendly
Bok choy, cooked (1 cup)	Calcium: 160 mg Vitamin K: 58 mcg	Good calcium absorption; low-calorie and versatile
Kale, cooked (1 cup)	Calcium: 180 mg Vitamin K: 1,060 mcg	Good calcium absorption; also provides magnesium; available fresh or frozen
Mustard greens, cooked (1 cup)	Calcium: 165 mg Vitamin K: 830 mcg	Peppery flavor; nutritional powerhouse that also provides vitamin A and C
Turnip greens, cooked (1 cup)	Calcium: 200 mg Vitamin K: 530 mcg	Often overlooked, but an excellent choice
Okra, cooked (1 cup)	Calcium: 120 mg Magnesium: 90 mg	Also provides vitamin K and folate; excellent absorption
Broccoli, cooked (1 cup)	Calcium: 60 mg Vitamin K: 220 mcg	Good calcium absorption; also provides vitamin C and other antioxidants

VEGETABLES AND LEAFY GREENS: LOWER ABSORPTION (HIGH OXALATE)

Food and Serving Size	Key Nutrients	Additional Notes
Spinach (1 cup cooked)	Calcium: 245 mg (only ~5% absorbed)	High oxalate content limits calcium absorption; still nutritious for other reasons (iron, vitamins), but not a reliable calcium source; same issue with Swiss chard and beet greens

Did You Know? Your body absorbs calcium from kale (41%) and collard greens (50%) better than from milk (32%). But not all greens are equal. Spinach, despite being "high in calcium," delivers only about 5% to your bones, because compounds called oxalates bind the calcium and block absorption.[59,60] Choose your greens wisely.

NUTS, SEEDS, AND HEALTHY FATS

Almonds, almond butter, chia seeds, sesame seeds/tahini, and Brazil nuts all provide calcium along with other bone-supporting nutrients.

Food and Serving Size	Key Nutrients	Additional Notes
Almonds (1 oz, about 23 nuts)	Calcium: 75 mg Protein: 6 g Magnesium: 75 mg	Vitamin E and healthy fats; portable and shelf-stable
Almond butter (2 tablespoons)	Calcium: 85 mg Protein: 7 g Magnesium: 90 mg	Now commonly available and a great substitute for peanut butter
Pumpkin seeds (pepitas) (1 oz)	Magnesium: 150 mg Zinc: 2 mg Protein: 8 g	One of the best plant sources of magnesium; also provides iron and healthy fats
Walnuts (1 oz)	Omega-3s (ALA): 2.5 g Magnesium: 45 mg	Excellent for reducing inflammation, which supports bone health
Chia seeds (2 tablespoons)	Calcium: 180 mg Protein: 4 g Omega-3 fatty acids (ALA): 5 g	Can be added to smoothies, yogurt, or oatmeal
Flaxseeds, ground (2 tbsp)	Omega-3s (ALA): 3 g Magnesium: 55 mg	Must be ground for body to absorb nutrients; easy to add to oatmeal or yogurt
Sesame seeds/tahini (2 tbsp)	Calcium: 130 mg (whole) or 65 mg (tahini)	Also provide magnesium and zinc; unhulled sesame seeds have much more calcium than hulled
Brazil nuts (1 oz, about 6 nuts)	Selenium: ~544 mcg (989% of the daily recommended value)—one of the richest food sources of selenium on Earth Magnesium: 105 mg	Also provide calcium and protein; limit to 1–2 nuts daily due to very high selenium content

FORTIFIED FOODS AND WHOLE GRAINS

Food and Serving Size	Key Nutrients	Additional Notes
Fortified breakfast cereals	250–1,000 mg calcium per serving (varies)	Often fortified with vitamin D; check labels, as fortification varies dramatically by brand
Fortified orange juice (1 cup)	Calcium: 300–350 mg Vitamin D: often 100 IU	Vitamin C enhances calcium absorption; shake well before pouring, as calcium settles at the bottom
Oatmeal, instant fortified (1 pkt)	Calcium: 100–150 mg	Also provides magnesium; choose plain varieties and add your own fruit to control sugar
Amaranth, cooked (1 cup)	Calcium: 116 mg Magnesium: 160 mg	An ancient grain (technically a seed) with unusually high calcium; nutty flavor
Teff, cooked (1 cup)	Calcium: 123 mg Magnesium: 126 mg	The grain used in Ethiopian injera bread; excellent calcium source for a grain
Whole grain bread, fortified (1 slice)	Calcium: 50–150 mg	Fortification varies, so check labels; also provides other nutrients and fiber

OTHER BONE-SUPPORTING FOODS

Food and Serving Size	Key Nutrients	Additional Notes
Prunes/dried plums (5–6 prunes)	Vitamin K, boron, and trace minerals	Research shows prunes may help prevent bone loss; they also support digestive health
Blackstrap molasses (1 tbsp)	Calcium: 200 mg Magnesium: 40 mg Iron: 3.5 mg	A traditional bone-builder; significantly higher nutrients than regular molasses; strong, bitter-sweet flavor
Kiwi (1 medium)	Vitamin K: 30 mcg Vitamin C: 64 mg	Vitamin C is essential for collagen formation in bone; very high vitamin C content per calorie
Figs, dried (¼ cup)	Calcium: 60 mg	Also provide magnesium and potassium; natural sweetness for snacks or cooking
Mushrooms (UV exposed, 3 oz)	Vitamin D: up to 400 IU	Must be UV exposed; most commercial mushrooms have minimal vitamin D unless specifically treated, so check the packaging
Natto (fermented soybeans) (3 oz)	Vitamin K2: 850 mcg Calcium: 100 mg Protein: 15 g	Acquired taste, but one of the richest food sources of vitamin K2

Did You Know? In a year-long clinical trial, postmenopausal women who ate just four to six prunes daily preserved hip bone density, while women who didn't eat prunes continued to lose bone. Researchers believe prunes' anti-inflammatory and antioxidant compounds help protect bone.[61]

FOODS TO LIMIT FOR BONE HEALTH

While focusing on adding bone-healthy foods is most important, it's also worth being aware of foods and beverages that can undermine your bone health efforts.

Food/Beverage to Limit	Impact on Bone Health	Guidelines and Better Alternatives
Excessive caffeine	>3–4 cups daily can increase calcium excretion	If you drink coffee heavily, ensure adequate calcium intake and consider cutting back gradually
Cola and soft drinks (including diet)	Phosphoric acid can disrupt calcium-phosphorus balance	Better choices: water, sparkling water with lemon, or herbal tea
Ultra-processed foods	Phosphate additives in baked goods, processed meats, and frozen meals may negatively affect calcium balance	Check labels for "phosphate" or "phosphoric acid"; choose minimally processed foods
Excessive alcohol	>2–3 drinks daily interferes with bone formation	Moderate consumption (1 drink/day for women, 1–2 for men) appears safe
Excessive salt	High sodium increases calcium excretion	Mainly a concern with processed foods; limit ultra-processed items

PUTTING IT TOGETHER: A DAY OF BONE-HEALTHY EATING

Here's what a day of solid bone-supporting meals might look like:

- **Breakfast:** Greek yogurt parfait with berries, almonds, and chia seeds. Coffee (limit to 1–2 cups). Provides calcium, protein, vitamin D, magnesium.
- **Lunch:** Salmon salad with mixed greens, including kale. Whole grain bread. Provides calcium, vitamin D, protein, vitamin K.
- **Snack:** Handful of almonds or almond butter with apple slices. Provides calcium, protein, magnesium.
- **Dinner/supper:** Grilled chicken or tofu. Steamed collard greens or broccoli. Quinoa or brown rice. Provides protein, calcium, vitamin K, trace minerals.
- **Evening:** Small serving of cheese with whole grain crackers, or dairy milk or fortified plant milk if needed to reach calcium goals.

This super-healthy sample eating plan provides roughly 1,000–1,200 mg calcium from food alone, along with substantial protein and other bone-supporting nutrients. You can adjust it based on your preferences, dietary restrictions, and supplement routine.

Remember: The goal isn't perfection at every meal but rather building a consistent pattern of including bone-healthy foods throughout your week. Focus on variety, emphasize whole foods, and let your food choices work alongside your exercise routine and any medications to build the strongest possible foundation for your bones.

EATING FOR BONE HEALTH WITH INFLAMMATORY OR AUTOIMMUNE DISEASES

Remember that for some people, osteoporosis is linked to another condition, like celiac disease or rheumatoid arthritis. Bone health benefits when these diseases are well-managed, which may be supported by a special diet. If you avoid gluten or eat a diet designed to decrease inflammation, keep doing that! Use the dietary information in this chapter as a way to tweak your diet to include more bone-building nutrients, not to totally change it from one that addresses what could be a root cause of your osteoporosis.

A HEALTHIER AND HAPPIER RELATIONSHIP WITH FOOD

About eight months into my nutritional overhaul, I realized my relationship with food had fundamentally changed. I no longer thought of meals as just fuel or comfort; food had become medicine and building materials for my skeletal reconstruction project.

Every glass of fortified almond milk, every serving of Greek yogurt, every handful of almonds represented an investment in my future strength and independence. The choices felt empowering rather than restrictive, because I understood exactly how they were helping my body heal and rebuild.

The approach was about making consistently better choices that supported my bone health goals, not following a "perfect" diet. Some days, I still craved diet cola or grabbed convenient processed foods, but these became occasional exceptions rather than daily habits.

As I focused on fueling my body properly and began to see improvements in my strength and energy, I knew there was one more piece of the puzzle to consider. While lifestyle changes were crucial, my FRAXplus score (remember that fracture risk calculator from Chapter 4?) suggested I needed more help to rebuild my bone bank. It was time to explore the world of osteoporosis medications.

KEY TAKEAWAYS

- Bone health requires multiple nutrients working together: calcium (1,200 mg daily for women over 50), vitamin D3 (1,000–2,000 IU daily for those with a deficiency), vitamin K2, magnesium, and adequate protein.
- Your body can only absorb about 500 mg of calcium at once, so split your intake throughout the day and take it separately from caffeine.
- Whole foods provide superior nutrition compared to supplements alone; focus on dairy, leafy greens, fatty fish, nuts, and adequate protein at every meal.

CHAPTER 9

MEDICATION CHOICES

Bisphosphonates, Anabolic Therapies, Hormonal Therapies, and Finding the Right Treatment

As I worked through my exercise program and focused on improving my nutrition during my months of recovery, I knew there was one more crucial decision ahead: medication. With four compression fractures at once and my FRAXplus score showing a major fracture risk (as discussed in Chapter 4), my doctor was adamant that I needed pharmaceutical reinforcement to rebuild my bone bank. I realize that many people resist medication, but for me, the question wasn't whether to take medication but which one would work best for my situation. I wanted to do everything I could to prevent future fractures.

I'll admit, the idea of daily medication felt daunting initially. As a physician, I knew the importance of evidence-based treatment, but as a patient, I found myself hoping that diet and exercise alone might be enough. Unfortunately, when your bone bank is as depleted as mine was (enough to cause multiple fractures), lifestyle changes alone often aren't sufficient. That's where osteoporosis medications come in. They're powerful tools designed to either slow withdrawals or accelerate deposits in your skeletal vault.

If your DEXA scan shows osteopenia rather than osteoporosis, you might be tempted to skip this chapter. Don't. As I mentioned in Chapter 4, my own T-scores showed "only" osteopenia, yet I had four compression fractures. That's because a low-impact fracture changes the equation: osteopenia plus fracture equals osteoporosis, regardless of what the numbers say. Your FRAX score, not just your T-score, determines whether medication makes sense for you. So, if you've already had a fracture, or if your fracture risk calculation puts you above the treatment threshold, this chapter is very much for you.

GETTING THE MOST OUT OF THIS CHAPTER

There's no way around it: covering all of the current osteoporosis medications well is going to get clinical. It's going to involve some tables and lists that may not seem important or interesting at first read. If it seems overwhelming, I suggest that you start by just skimming to learn about how these medicines work. Save any dive into the tables for if and when you need to have detailed conversations with your doctor.

UNDERSTANDING HOW THESE MEDICATIONS WORK

Think of osteoporosis medications as different types of managers for your bone bank, each with their own approach to protecting and rebuilding bone strength.

The most common kinds of osteoporosis medicine are known as **antiresorptive medications**. They work like careful financial advisers, putting the brakes on excessive withdrawals from your bone account. These medications include bisphosphonates like alendronate (Fosamax), risedronate (Actonel), and zoledronic acid (Reclast or Zometa), along with denosumab (Prolia). They slow down the osteoclasts (remember those bone-demolition cells from Chapter 3?), telling them to take a coffee break.

Anabolic medications function more like aggressive investment strategies, stimulating new bone formation by encouraging osteoblasts to work overtime. These include teriparatide (Forteo), abaloparatide (Tymlos), and romosozumab (Evenity). Think of them as bringing in extra construction crews to rapidly build new deposits in your bone bank.

Hormonal therapies like raloxifene (Evista) or estrogen work more gently, helping to maintain the delicate balance between deposits and withdrawals. These are particularly useful for postmenopausal women who have lost estrogen's protective effects.

BENEFITS VS. RISKS OF MEDICATIONS

I've included information on any side effects associated with the medications I discuss in this chapter. Each one has risks, and it's important to talk to your medical provider and weigh the risks against the benefits in your particular situation.

In most cases, the serious side effects are exceedingly rare. So, keep an open mind. Don't let the fear of rare side effects stop you from even considering medication that could prevent fractures stealing away years of active life.

ANTIRESORPTIVE MEDICATIONS

Bisphosphonates: The Proven Workhorses

Bisphosphonates represent the most commonly prescribed osteoporosis medications, and their track record justifies this popularity. They're effective, extensively studied, and now available in affordable generic formulations that make treatment accessible to most patients.

The flexibility in how you can take them was appealing to me initially. Alendronate (Fosamax) comes as daily or weekly pills; risedronate (Actonel) offers daily, weekly, or monthly options; ibandronate (Boniva) can be taken as a tablet monthly or given as a quarterly IV infusion; and zoledronic acid (Reclast) requires only an annual IV treatment. For someone with a busy schedule, less frequent dosing seemed attractive.

The effectiveness numbers are impressive. These medications reduce vertebral fractures by 40–70% and hip fractures by 40–50%, with meaningful reductions in other fracture types as well. This is substantial protection that can preserve independence and quality of life for most people.[62,63]

If you end up taking an oral bisphosphonate, the instructions are crucial but admittedly inconvenient. You must take it first thing in the morning on an empty stomach with a full glass of plain water, then stay upright for at least 30–60 minutes before eating, drinking anything else, or lying down. This prevents the medication from irritating your esophagus and helps your body absorb it properly.

Understanding the side effects is reassuring for most people. Serious side effects are uncommon. The most common issues involve stomach upset with oral forms of the medication and flu-like symptoms after IV infusions. Two rare but serious concerns with long-term use are osteonecrosis (death of bone) inside the jaw, which is more common in people receiving high-dose IV bisphosphonates for cancer or those who undergo teeth extraction, and atypical femur fractures, which are unusual breaks in the thigh bone. Both are very rare in people taking standard doses for osteoporosis. Osteonecrosis of the jaw has been reported in 1 in 100,000 to 1 in 1,000 patients, with the higher rates seen in long-term users (see Did You Know? box). This helps to explain why some doctors recommend a "drug holiday" after several years of treatment.[64]

Medication and Usage	Mechanism and Side Effects	Important Notes
Alendronate (Fosamax, Fosavance, Vantavo) **Pill**: Daily or weekly **Cost**: Low	**Action**: Slows osteoclast activity; preserves existing bone. **Side effects**: Heartburn, stomach upset, esophageal irritation. Rare: jaw problems, unusual thigh fractures.	Generic available. Must take on empty stomach and stay upright for 30–60 minutes. Reduces both vertebral and hip fractures by 40–50%.65
Risedronate (Actonel, Atelvia) **Pill**: Daily, weekly, or monthly **Cost**: Low	**Action**: Slows osteoclast activity. **Side effects**: Like alendronate, but may have slightly less gastrointestinal (GI) upset.	Generic available; flexible dosing. Similar efficacy and administration rules to alendronate.

Medication and Usage	Mechanism and Side Effects	Important Notes
Ibandronate (Bonviva, Bondronat, Bondenza) **Pill**: Monthly **IV**: Every 3 months **Cost**: Low to medium	**Action**: Slows osteoclast activity. **Side effects**: Pill: Similar GI effects to alendronate. IV: Flu-like symptoms for 1–3 days post-infusion.	Less frequent dosing. IV form avoids GI side effects. Proven benefit mainly for spine fractures.
Zoledronic acid (Reclast, Aclasta, Zometa) **IV infusion**: Once yearly **Cost**: Medium	**Action**: Slows osteoclast activity. **Side effects**: Flu-like symptoms (fever, aches) 1–3 days after first dose. Rare: kidney problems.	Convenient yearly dosing. No GI side effects. Requires adequate hydration and kidney monitoring. Very effective for all fracture types, with up to a 70% reduction in vertebral fractures.

Did You Know? If you're worried about jaw problems with bisphosphonates, here's some perspective. For patients taking oral bisphosphonates at osteoporosis doses, the risk of osteonecrosis of the jaw has been estimated at anywhere from 1 in 100,000 to 1 in 1,000. That's a wide range, and it deserves a brief explanation. The lowest estimates come from early data and spontaneous reports. The highest come from a large study that specifically looked at patients who had been taking oral bisphosphonates for four or more years, which is the population most relevant to you, since these medications are meant for long-term use. Even at the higher end of that range, the risk remains very low: roughly 1 in 1,000 patients. Most cases occur in cancer patients receiving IV doses that are hundreds of times higher than those used for osteoporosis treatment.[66,67,68,69]

Denosumab: A Different Approach

Denosumab (Prolia) offers an alternative: a simple injection just under the skin every six months that blocks the signals telling bone cells to break down. The advantages include ease of use (since you get it at the doctor's office), no stomach upset, and highly effective bone density improvements.

The potential downsides of denosumab include the potential for low blood calcium levels (after all, bone breakdown is the body's way of rapidly increasing blood calcium levels), especially in people with kidney problems, and the need for careful planning around any treatment discontinuation. Stopping denosumab suddenly can lead to rapid bone loss, so transitions to other medications require careful timing and monitoring.

Medication and Usage	Mechanism and Side Effects	Important Notes
Denosumab (Prolia, Xgeva) **Injection**: Every 6 months **Cost**: Medium to high	**Action**: Blocks signals that activate osteoclasts. **Side effects**: Low calcium, skin infections, back/muscle pain. Rare: jaw problems, unusual thigh fractures.	No stomach issues. Excellent bone density improvements. Cannot stop abruptly (rapid bone loss occurs). Must transition to another drug if stopping.

ANABOLIC MEDICATIONS: THE HEAVY ARTILLERY

For people at extremely high fracture risk (like me, with my multiple existing fractures), anabolic medications can provide game-changing bone-building power. These medications represent the most potent tools available for severely depleted bone banks.

Generic teriparatide became my choice after careful consideration with my doctor. It requires a daily injection that I give myself, usually in my belly, using a pen device similar to the one people with diabetes use for insulin. The needle is genuinely tiny. It's much smaller than the one used to give you a vaccine. After the first few days, the injection became just part of my routine. At first, I took it at bedtime, but I've since switched to mornings, as recent studies have indicated it may be more effective when taken early in the day.

What makes these bone-building medications special is their unique ability to build new bone rather than just prevent loss. The fracture prevention results are impressive. Both teriparatide (Forteo) and abaloparatide (Tymlos) work remarkably well; in one major head-to-head study, they reduced new vertebral fractures by approximately 80–86%, with meaningful reductions in non-vertebral fractures as well. When compared directly against standard medications like bisphosphonates, these bone-builders prove superior.[70,71]

Romosozumab (Evenity) is another powerful option for people at very high fracture risk. Compared with no treatment, romosozumab cut spine fractures by nearly three-quarters after just one year. In studies comparing it directly against a standard bisphosphonate, it still showed significantly better results across all fracture types.[72,73]

For someone who's already fractured, these results go beyond statistics; they represent the difference between maintaining independence and facing another devastating fracture. These medications also build substantial new bone, with density increases that can take years to achieve with other treatments.

An unexpected bonus I discovered was that teriparatide is associated with reduced back pain from vertebral fractures. About two months after starting treatment, I noticed a significant improvement in the chronic back pain I'd been living with since my fractures. I hadn't expected this. The pain relief was a welcome surprise that improved my quality of life beyond just the bone-building benefits.

That doesn't mean that the reality of daily injections wasn't initially scary. Giving myself a shot every day seemed overwhelming, but the pen device makes the process foolproof. Most days, I barely feel the injection. The knowledge that each tiny shot is actively rebuilding my bone strength makes it feel empowering rather than burdensome.

I'll be taking teriparatide for another year or two from the time of this writing. Anabolic medications used to have a firm two-year lifetime use restriction based on early studies in rats, but this limitation was removed by the FDA in November 2020 after real-world evidence showed no increased cancer risk in humans. However, most treatment courses still last 18–24 months, as this represents the time frame for optimal bone-building benefit. The important consideration is that anabolic medications work best when followed by antiresorptive therapy to maintain the bone gains achieved. Without this follow-up treatment, much of the benefit can be lost over time.

Medication and Usage	Mechanism and Side Effects	Important Notes
Teriparatide (Forteo, Forsteo) **Daily self-injection** **Cost**: Very high	**Action**: Stimulates osteoblasts; actively builds new bone. **Side effects**: Nausea, leg cramps, dizziness. Temporary high calcium levels.	Most potent bone-builder. Increases spine density significantly. Treatment typically 18–24 months. Must follow with antiresorptive to maintain gains. Available as a generic with a modest reduction in cost.

Medication and Usage	Mechanism and Side Effects	Important Notes
Abaloparatide (Tymlos, Eladynos) Daily self-injection **Cost**: Very high	**Action**: Stimulates osteoblasts; actively builds new bone. **Side effects**: Dizziness, nausea, headache, palpitations.	Like teriparatide. Treatment limited to 2 years. Must follow with antiresorptive to maintain gains.
Romosozumab (Evenity) **Injection**: Monthly for 12 months **Cost**: Very high	**Action**: Dual-action: increases bone formation and decreases resorption. **Side effects**: Joint pain, headache. Caution: May increase risk of cardiac events.	Rapid density gains. Limited to 12 months. Reserved for those with very high risk. Not for recent heart attack/stroke patients. Must follow with antiresorptive.

HORMONAL TREATMENTS

Selective Estrogen Receptor Modulators: Raloxifene

Raloxifene (Evista) represents a different approach to bone protection, particularly for women who can't or prefer not to use traditional hormone replacement therapy. As a selective estrogen receptor modulator (or SERM), it acts like estrogen in some tissues (such as bones) while blocking estrogen effects in others (such as breasts). It's taken as a single daily pill, making compliance straightforward.[74]

The drug's selective action offers an interesting bonus beyond bone protection: it reduces the risk of invasive breast cancer by 35% or more, similar to what we see with tamoxifen (a SERM used in the treatment of some breast cancers). For women with a family history of breast cancer who also need bone protection, this dual benefit can be particularly appealing.[75]

However, raloxifene's bone effects are more modest than those of bisphosphonates or anabolic medications. It reduces vertebral fractures by about 35%, but it hasn't shown clear benefit for hip fractures.

The downsides include hot flashes, which can be problematic for women still experiencing menopausal symptoms, and an increased risk of blood clots (similar to estrogen therapy). Leg cramps are another common complaint; some women find these bothersome enough that they discontinue treatment.

Medication and Usage	Mechanism and Side Effects	Important Notes
Raloxifene (Evista) **Pill:** Daily **Cost:** Low to medium	**Action:** Acts like estrogen in bones; blocks estrogen in breast tissues. **Side effects:** Hot flashes, leg cramps, increased blood clot risk.	Reduces vertebral fractures ~35% (no proven hip benefit). Bonus: Reduces breast cancer risk ~35%. Not for women with hot flashes.76

Hormone Replacement Therapy: Effect on Bones

When I explored the possibility of hormone replacement therapy (HRT) after my diagnosis, I discovered that the story around HRT and bone health is more nuanced than I'd initially understood. HRT effectively reduces fracture risk across the skeleton by approximately 20–40% depending on the fracture type, making it one of the most comprehensive bone-protective treatments available; however, its role in osteoporosis treatment has become complicated by concerns about other health risks.

The Women's Health Initiative study, published in 2002, fundamentally changed how doctors and patients think about HRT. The study revealed increased risks of breast cancer, heart disease, and blood clots with long-term use, leading to dramatic declines in HRT prescriptions. However, subsequent analyses have shown that the benefit–risk balance depends heavily on individual factors: when HRT is started (earlier is safer), the type of hormones used, the dose, and how the medication is delivered.[77]

For bone health specifically, HRT works by replacing estrogen, whose levels plummets during menopause. Since estrogen helps maintain the balance between bone breakdown and bone building, restoring estrogen levels can effectively slow bone loss. What makes HRT unique among osteoporosis treatments is that it's the only medication proven to reduce fracture risk regardless of your baseline fracture probability. Whether you're at low, moderate, or elevated risk, HRT provides measurable bone protection.[78]

The challenge with HRT for bone health is that its benefits disappear once you stop taking it. Unlike bisphosphonates, which can provide residual protection for years after you discontinue treatment, stopping HRT means your bones resume the accelerated loss pattern typical of untreated menopause. Think of it like maintaining a garden: HRT keeps your bone health flourishing while you're using it, but if you stop watering the garden, it quickly wilts.

Current guidelines suggest HRT should be considered primarily for women experiencing significant menopausal symptoms (hot flashes, night sweats, vaginal dryness) who also need bone protection. For someone dealing with debilitating hot flashes anyway, adding bone protection may be a welcome bonus rather than the primary goal. The recommendation is to use the lowest effective dose for the shortest time needed.

For me personally, while HRT might have helped my bones, my cardiovascular risk factors and family history made it a less appealing choice. I didn't have significant menopausal symptoms that would have tipped the balance in HRT's favor. But I recognize that for many women, and particularly those who start HRT around menopause for symptom relief, the bone-protective effects represent important added value.

If you're considering HRT, the conversation with your doctor should include your individual risk factors for breast cancer, heart disease, and blood clots, as well as the severity of your menopausal symptoms and your fracture risk. The decision is highly personal and needs you to weigh multiple factors unique to your situation.

Medication and Usage	Mechanism and Side Effects	Important Notes
Hormone replacement therapy (HRT) **Pill, patch, or cream:** Daily **Cost:** Low	**Action:** Replaces estrogen to maintain bone balance. **Side effects:** Breast tenderness, bloating. Risks: Clots, stroke, heart disease.	Reduces all fractures by 20–40%. Only drug effective at all risk levels. Benefits stop when medication stops. Best for women with menopausal symptoms.79

Calcitonin: A Treatment Largely Left Behind

You might come across calcitonin in your research about osteoporosis medications, so it's worth understanding why this once-popular treatment has fallen out of favor. Calcitonin is a hormone that's naturally produced by your thyroid gland that helps regulate calcium levels. Synthetic versions (usually derived from salmon, because it's more potent than human calcitonin) were once commonly prescribed as nasal sprays or injections.

The medication works by temporarily inhibiting osteoclasts, those bone-demolition cells we discussed in Chapter 4. In theory, slowing down the demolition crew should help preserve bone. However, the reality proved disappointing. Large studies have shown that calcitonin only modestly reduces vertebral fractures and provides no clear benefit for hip fractures or other non-spine fractures. Compared to bisphosphonates or other modern treatments, calcitonin's bone-protective effects are substantially weaker.

A bigger concern emerged when long-term studies revealed a small but measurable increase in cancer risk with extended calcitonin use, particularly the nasal spray formulation. The risk increase was small, but, when combined with the medication's limited effectiveness, it meant that the benefit–risk balance no longer made sense for most patients. Many countries, including Canada and much of Europe, withdrew the nasal spray formulation from their markets.[80]

In the United States, calcitonin remains FDA-approved, but it's less often prescribed for osteoporosis these days. One scenario where some doctors still consider it is for acute pain relief following vertebral compression fractures. Some patients report that calcitonin helps with the severe back pain these fractures can cause, though the evidence for this benefit is mixed.

If you're currently taking calcitonin for osteoporosis, it's worth discussing with your doctor whether more effective alternatives might be appropriate for you.

Medication and Usage	Mechanism and Side Effects	Important Notes
Calcitonin Nasal spray or injection **Cost:** Low	**Action:** Temporarily inhibits osteoclasts. **Side effects:** Nasal irritation, nausea, flushing.	Rarely used. Modest spine benefit only. Small potential cancer risk with long-term use. Less effective than other options.

SEQUENTIAL TREATMENT STRATEGY

Understanding the importance of treatment sequencing became crucial in my decision-making. Bone-building medications work powerfully, but stopping them without transitioning to a bone-preserving medication can result in rapid bone loss, meaning you lose much of what you've gained. Research also suggests that the opposite approach (using a bone-preserving medication before a bone-building one) may limit how much new bone the builder can create.

This is why treatment planning often involves starting with bone-building therapy for high-risk patients, then transitioning to bone-preserving antiresorptive medication to lock in the benefits. If needed, your doctor will help determine the optimal timing and sequence based on your individual situation.

MAKING MY TREATMENT DECISION

As I mentioned earlier in the section on anabolic medications, I chose to take generic teriparatide. My FRAXplus score of 22%, which was above the 20% threshold that typically triggers treatment recommendations, and my recent multiple vertebral fractures meant I was able to secure insurance approval for it.

I carefully considered other options during my decision-making process. Having gone through hysterectomy at 47, I revisited the possibility of HRT. Research shows that it can provide some bone benefits, but my cardiovascular risk factors and family history made this option less appealing for me personally.

The decision felt empowering once I understood my options fully. It represented a choice to actively rebuild what I'd lost and invest in my future independence; it wasn't simply about taking medication.

UNDERSTANDING REALISTIC TIMELINES

Setting appropriate expectations helped me stay motivated as I started my treatment. Anabolic medications like teriparatide work quickly, with measurable bone density improvements often visible within six months and peak effects typically reached by 18–24 months.

Bisphosphonates work more gradually, with meaningful bone density increases usually developing over one to three years of consistent use. The maximum fracture risk reduction often takes two to three years to achieve, though some protection begins earlier.

Follow-up DEXA scans typically take place one to two years after starting treatment to assess response. A gain of 3% or more in bone density is considered meaningful improvement, though even smaller gains combined with fracture risk reduction represent treatment success.

I had to adjust my expectations about returning to "normal" bone density. The goal is stabilizing or improving what you have and significantly reducing fracture risk, not necessarily getting back to what you had at age 30.

LIVING WITH DAILY TREATMENT

My daily medication routine has evolved into something much more meaningful than simple medication compliance. As I prepare the pen and find a spot on my belly, I often reflect on the previous day's choices: Did I get adequate calcium from my food? Did I do my exercises? Did I choose milk or water over my old vice, diet cola?

That little injection has become a daily reminder that I'm actively fighting for my bone health rather than passively accepting weakness. The needle goes in, barely perceptible, and I know I've just made another deposit in my bone bank. Tomorrow, my osteoblasts will receive the signal to keep building. Tomorrow, I'll be incrementally stronger than today.

Understanding that this small daily action contributes to measurable bone building has transformed what could feel like medical drudgery into an empowering ritual of self-care and investment in my future.

THE LONG-TERM COMMITMENT

Just as bone-building exercise and a calcium-rich diet need to be lifelong to be effective, osteoporosis medications usually require long-term commitment. Osteoporosis and osteopenia aren't conditions you cure and move on from; they're something you manage actively, like blood pressure or high cholesterol. But that commitment can feel empowering when you frame it properly.

Every pill taken, every exercise class completed, and every doctor's appointment attended represents a choice you're making for your future self. You're choosing strength over fragility and proactive health management over passive acceptance.

Taking control of my bone health through medication wasn't about preventing future fractures; it was about reclaiming my sense of agency over my body. But medication, exercise, and nutrition were only part of my journey. Working effectively with my healthcare team became essential for managing the complexities of treatment decisions and long-term management.

KEY TAKEAWAYS

- Osteoporosis medications work in different ways: antiresorptive drugs (like bisphosphonates) slow bone breakdown, while anabolic medications actively stimulate new bone formation.
- Bisphosphonates are the most prescribed and well-studied option, with proven effectiveness in reducing fracture risk by 40–70% depending on the type of fracture.
- Managing osteoporosis is a long-term commitment, like treating blood pressure or cholesterol; consistent treatment and monitoring are essential for maintaining bone strength.

CHAPTER 10

WORKING WITH YOUR HEALTHCARE TEAM

Finding Specialists, Asking Questions, and Advocating for Yourself

After my diagnosis, I realized that managing osteoporosis effectively would require more than just my own efforts; I needed the right medical team to support me. As a physician myself, I had advantages when it came to working through the healthcare system, but I also discovered that not all medical providers approach bone health with the same level of expertise or urgency. Learning to advocate for appropriate care became an essential skill, even with my medical background.

Getting optimal osteoporosis care often requires being an informed and persistent advocate for yourself. The complexity of bone health assessment, the variety of treatment options, and the long-term nature of management mean that finding the right healthcare partners can make the difference between thriving and simply surviving with this condition.

FINDING THE RIGHT SPECIALISTS

While primary care providers can manage straightforward osteoporosis, complex cases often benefit from specialist expertise. When I needed approval for my expensive anabolic medication, having a doctor familiar with FRAXplus scoring as well as insurance requirements made all the difference.

Ideally, anyone with severe osteoporosis or multiple fractures would have access to a major medical center with a dedicated osteoporosis clinic that brings together specialists from multiple disciplines. These comprehensive programs offer advanced testing options and coordinated care approaches that can be particularly valuable.

> **Did You Know?** Hospitals with dedicated bone health programs reduce the risk of a second fracture by about 40%. These coordinated care teams bring together specialists who ensure patients get proper evaluation and treatment. If your hospital has one, ask for a referral. If not, you may need to build that team yourself.[81]

In my case, a physiatrist (a physical medicine and rehabilitation doctor) made my diagnosis. Physiatrists specialize in treating a wide variety of conditions related to musculoskeletal and neurological impairments. My physiatrist's experience with disorders of the spine was helpful, and I'm grateful that she really listened when I showed up in pain and immediately ordered that first MRI.

Endocrinologists (hormone specialists) who specialize in bone health bring deep expertise in hormonal factors affecting bones alongside experience with the full range of available medications. They're often the best choice for complex cases involving multiple risk factors or previous treatment failures. I didn't see an endocrinologist simply because I already had a relationship with a rheumatologist who specialized in osteoporosis.

Rheumatologists (inflammatory and autoimmune disease specialists) with osteoporosis expertise understand the intricate relationships between inflammatory diseases and bone health. They're particularly valuable for patients whose bone loss relates to autoimmune conditions or long-term steroid use, which are situations where both the underlying disease and its treatment affect bone health.

Orthopedists (bone and joint specialists; often, these are surgeons) sometimes specialize in metabolic bone disease, especially those who work in fracture prevention clinics. These specialists understand both the medical management and surgical implications of severe osteoporosis, which can be invaluable if you're dealing with complex fractures. You'll be working with an orthopedist if you need surgical treatment for a broken hip or vertebra.

If you've suffered painful fractures, it's essential to have a pain management doctor on your team. Mine not only managed my pain medicine but also monitored my MRIs for healing and fitted me for a specialized back brace. He and his physician assistant had experience of treating people with compression fractures, and they gave me reassurance that my long healing process wasn't unusual.

Finally, including a counselor on your team is invaluable if you struggle with anxiety or depression about your diagnosis. It's a lot to deal with emotionally, and you don't need to go through it on your own.

PREPARING FOR YOUR APPOINTMENTS

Productive osteoporosis consultations require preparation, and I learned this even as a physician seeking care. Gather your complete medical history, including all medications you've taken but especially steroids (even short courses for things like poison ivy or severe asthma). Include any previous fractures, even minor ones, any height loss you may have noticed, family history of osteoporosis or fractures, and an honest assessment of lifestyle factors like smoking, alcohol use, and exercise habits.

Most importantly, bring copies of any previous DEXA scans, not just the most recent report. Trends over time provide crucial information that specialists need for optimal decision-making. I've seen too many patients who only have their latest report, which means they miss the opportunity to see patterns of bone loss or stability that could influence treatment choices.

If you've had other relevant testing, such as blood work for vitamin D levels or tests for secondary causes of bone loss, include those results as well. The more complete picture you can provide, the better your specialist can tailor your care.

ESSENTIAL QUESTIONS TO ASK

Come prepared with specific questions that will help you understand your situation and treatment options. Don't accept vague reassurances. Ask for your exact T-scores and Z-scores from DEXA scans. Request your 10-year fracture risk calculation using both standard FRAX and FRAXplus if available.

Inquire about whether you're a candidate for TBS analysis to assess your bone quality beyond density. This was helpful in my case, as my borderline TBS helped explain why I fractured despite having only osteopenia rather than full osteoporosis.

Talk about non-pharmaceutical options. Is your fracture risk low enough that you could safely try a diet and exercise program before taking any medication? That is always preferable, but, quite honestly, sometimes doctors can be cynical about the chances of patients being able to make (and sustain) big changes in their lifestyles. Don't take it personally. If your doctor doesn't think you need medication, or you decline medication, be sure to *schedule a repeat DEXA scan in one year* to see if your diet and exercise changes are effective.

If medicine is recommended, ask specifically about the reasoning behind medication choice: why one drug over another, what the expected timeline for benefits looks like, and how treatment response will be monitored. Understanding the "why" behind recommendations helps you make informed decisions and stay motivated during treatment.

Don't hesitate to ask about side effects: both the serious rare ones and the common minor ones that might affect your daily life. Understanding what to expect helps you distinguish normal adjustment periods from concerning symptoms that warrant medical attention.

ADVOCATING FOR APPROPRIATE TESTING

Not all healthcare providers stay current with advances in bone health assessment. If your doctor seems unfamiliar with FRAX-plus or TBS analysis, it's reasonable to ask whether these tools might provide valuable information for your case. Blood testing for "bone turnover markers" can sometimes be helpful, as the results provide information on the balance of bone formation vs. bone breakdown. While not needed in all cases, getting these additional assessments can sometimes mean the difference between qualifying for advanced treatments or not.

Similarly, if you have risk factors for secondary osteoporosis (osteoporosis due to another illness), make sure that appropriate testing for underlying causes has been done. Risk factors include inflammatory diseases, gut malabsorption issues, and endocrine (hormonal) disorders. Sometimes, treating an underlying condition can dramatically improve bone health outcomes.

Follow-up DEXA scanning is important. Any intervention aimed at improving bone health should be followed by repeat scanning to assess its effectiveness. The timing varies, but follow-up typically occurs one to two years after starting treatment. Don't let your doctor dismiss the need for monitoring; you need to know if your treatment is working.

UNDERSTANDING INSURANCE COVERAGE

Navigating insurance coverage for osteoporosis care in the U.S. requires patience and persistence. To advocate for yourself, you'll need to understand your coverage. If calling your insurance company isn't helpful, ask your employer for the "Summary Plan

Description" document that they're required to provide on request. If you're covered by Medicare or a state Medicaid program, you should be able to find information on their websites. For those with Medicare Advantage programs or Medicare Part D coverage, look for the "Evidence of Coverage" document online. These documents provide more detailed information on coverage.

In addition to understanding your insurance coverage for osteoporosis, I recommend scheduling an appointment with your primary healthcare provider (or specialist if you have one) specifically for bone health. Make sure the diagnoses on your record for the visit include one relating to your bones: osteoporosis, osteopenia, fragility, compression fractures (old or new), or even vitamin D deficiency. This way, if your doctor needs to submit information to your insurance company about your diagnosis, the record is easy to find. You may need to go through some hoops or even write appeal letters to get the most effective medications.

DEXA scans are well-covered, but age and frequency limitations may apply. Most plans cover scans every two years, though medical necessity can sometimes justify more frequent monitoring. If you or your doctor feel you need a DEXA scan but your insurance is refusing coverage even after an appeal, consider asking what the self-pay cost is for the scan. You can sometimes find prices as low as $150, and it would be eligible for reimbursement under most Health Savings Accounts.

Medication coverage varies dramatically between plans and specific drugs. Generic bisphosphonates usually have minimal copays, while newer medications may require prior authorization or step therapy protocols (trying and "failing" a medication, due to lack of effectiveness or side effects, before being eligible for another one). Your doctor's office can help with prior authorization paperwork, but having documentation of your FRAX or FRAXplus scores and any problems or side effects with first-line treatments strengthens approval chances for the more powerful (and more expensive) treatments.

If you can't tolerate an osteoporosis medication due to side effects, don't give up. Have your doctor document the side effects well, and you'll likely be able to try another medication, even if it's more expensive and requires a prior authorization from your insurance company.

Some insurance plans have specialty pharmacies for expensive medications like anabolic agents. These often provide additional support services, including injection training and adherence monitoring, which can improve treatment success. When I started teriparatide, the specialty pharmacy provided detailed injection training and monthly check-ins, which were invaluable.

WHEN TO SEEK A SECOND OPINION

Consider consulting another specialist if your current healthcare provider seems dismissive of your bone health concerns or unfamiliar with newer treatment options. I've seen too many patients whose doctors minimized their fracture concerns or suggested that age-related bone loss was inevitable and not worth addressing.

Similarly, if you're experiencing side effects that your doctor minimizes or if your bone density continues to decline despite treatment, a fresh perspective can be valuable. Sometimes, it feels awkward to get a second opinion, but suboptimal care can lead to a life-changing fracture.

BUILDING LONG-TERM PARTNERSHIPS

Osteoporosis management is a marathon, not a sprint. The relationships you build with your healthcare team will span years or decades, making compatibility and communication style important considerations. You want medical providers who listen to your concerns and respect your preferences while guiding you toward evidence-based care.

Regular communication between appointments helps address concerns before they become problems. Many practices have patient portals or nurse phone lines for questions about side effects, medication timing, or activity restrictions. Don't hesitate to use these resources when you need guidance.

RED FLAGS IN OSTEOPOROSIS CARE

Certain approaches should prompt you to seek care elsewhere. Doctors who dismiss fracture concerns in people with osteoporosis, who neglect to order follow-up DEXA scans after treatment initiation, or who suggest that calcium supplementation alone will reverse osteoporosis may not be providing optimal care.

Similarly, medical providers who seem unfamiliar with newer treatment options, or are uninterested in learning about them, may not have the expertise needed for complex bone health management.

THE IMPORTANCE OF TAKING BONE LOSS SERIOUSLY

One of the most crucial aspects of good osteoporosis care is working with medical providers who take bone loss seriously. Given the sobering statistics about fracture impacts, osteoporosis isn't just a normal part of aging; it's a medical condition with effective treatments that can significantly reduce fracture risk and preserve independence.

Your healthcare team should view fracture prevention as a priority worth pursuing actively, not a luxury to consider only after other health issues are addressed. The consequences of untreated osteoporosis, including loss of independence, chronic pain, and increased mortality risk, are too significant to ignore or minimize.

Finding healthcare providers who share your commitment to maintaining bone health creates the foundation for successful long-term management. With the right team in place, you can focus your energy on the lifestyle changes and treatment adherence that will keep you strong and active for years to come. But even with excellent medical care, daily life with osteoporosis requires some practical adjustments to stay safe while remaining active. Part 3 of this book addresses how to live well with osteoporosis.

KEY TAKEAWAYS

- Complex osteoporosis cases often benefit from specialist care. Endocrinologists and rheumatologists with bone health expertise can provide advanced treatment strategies.
- Be an active advocate for your health by asking specific questions about your bone density numbers, fracture risk scores, and treatment options.
- A good healthcare team takes bone health seriously as a priority; it doesn't treat it as something to address only after other conditions are managed.

PART 3

LIVING WELL WITH OSTEOPOROSIS

CHAPTER 11

LIVING SAFELY WITH OSTEOPOROSIS

Fall Prevention, Home Safety, and Staying Active

For me, one of the most challenging aspects of living with osteoporosis turned out to be finding the balance between reasonable caution and paralyzing fear. After my diagnosis, I became hyperaware of every potential fall risk and every activity that might put my fragile bones at risk. Learning to live safely without becoming a prisoner of my own anxiety required both practical strategies and significant emotional adjustment.

The goal isn't wrapping yourself in bubble wrap; that approach worsens bone health by promoting inactivity. Instead, it's about becoming more thoughtful about your environment and daily activities while maintaining the active, engaged lifestyle that supports both bone health and overall well-being.

Did You Know? About half of older adults experience fear of falling, and half of those people limit their activities because of that fear. But research shows that this creates a vicious cycle: avoiding activity leads to deconditioning, which actually increases your risk of falling.[82],[83] The goal isn't eliminating caution; it's channeling it into smart precautions while staying active.

UNDERSTANDING YOUR REAL RISKS

Fear is often greater than the actual risk when it comes to osteoporosis, and I fell into this trap initially. I found myself avoiding activities that were probably safe while overlooking genuinely risky situations. Understanding what truly increases fracture risk helped me make more informed decisions about which precautions mattered most.

Most osteoporotic fractures result from falls from standing height or less, not dramatic accidents or high-impact activities. This means that preventing everyday falls becomes your primary safety focus. The activities most likely to cause dangerous falls often aren't the ones people worry about most.

Falls most commonly occur during routine activities: getting up at night to use the bathroom, stepping off curbs, navigating stairs, or walking on uneven surfaces. Walking large, energetic dogs presents a particular risk that many people don't consider seriously enough. My experience with Finnegan taught me that a sudden lunge toward another dog, a squirrel, or an interesting smell can easily pull you off balance.

After my fractures, my husband, a little begrudgingly, took over most of Finnegan's walking duties. (Never promise your partner that you'll take care of all the dog-walking in order to get a puppy.) We eventually installed a fence in our backyard, which was a practical adaptation that preserved both my safety and the dog's exercise needs. These adjustments initially felt like admissions of weakness, but they were actually intelligent accommodations that preserved my independence in the areas that mattered most.

CREATING A SAFER HOME ENVIRONMENT

Your home environment significantly influences your fall risk, and most hazards can be modified easily and inexpensively. Lighting improvements provided some of the highest-impact changes for me. I made sure we had good lighting in all areas, especially pathways to bathrooms at night. Motion-activated night lights eliminated the need to fumble for switches in the dark.

I removed or secured area rugs, particularly those without non-slip backing. Even small throw rugs can create tripping hazards. If you want to keep rugs for comfort or aesthetics, use double-sided tape or non-slip backing to secure them completely.

When we'd moved into our home a decade earlier, it already had grab bars installed in both bathrooms by the toilet and in the shower, along with handrails on both sides of the staircase. We debated removing them initially, since they seemed "too early" for people in their 40s, but we ultimately decided to leave them, figuring that someday we'd need them. I hadn't realized how soon that day would come, but I'm incredibly grateful we kept them. They've already prevented several potential falls, including among younger members of the family, and now I believe all homes should have these safety features installed proactively rather than waiting until they're suddenly needed.

I cleared pathways of clutter and electrical cords that might cause tripping. I paid particular attention to the route from my bedroom to the bathroom, since nighttime navigation carries higher fall risk due to grogginess and reduced lighting.

SAFE MOVEMENT STRATEGIES

How you move through daily activities can significantly impact your fall risk. I learned to always allow extra time for activities, so I didn't feel rushed. Hurrying increases the likelihood of missed steps and inattention to hazards. No more rapid-fire run-through-the-house cleaning sessions before company. I plan ahead and ask my family to pitch in.

When getting up from my bed, I now sit on the edge for a moment before standing to avoid dizziness from position changes. I'm extra careful when walking in unfamiliar environments or when feeling unsteady.

I avoid carrying large loads that obstruct my vision or affect my balance. Making multiple trips rather than trying to carry everything at once became a new habit. When I have to carry items multiple things, I use a backpack or a bag that keeps my hands free for balance.

Stairs require special caution. I use handrails whenever I can, and I make sure each foot is securely placed before taking the next step. I try to avoid the stairs in the middle of the night, if I'm in a hurry, or if I'm carrying items that might affect my balance. Again, this means I sometimes need to ask my family for help. When that's hard for me to do, I just remind myself of the pain those compression fractures caused and how I have some power to avoid that happening again.

FOOTWEAR THAT PROTECTS

Proper footwear plays a crucial role in fall prevention. You don't necessarily need to start wearing old-fashioned orthopedic shoes. You do need to give some thought to how your shoes affect your balance and your fall risk.

Shoes should fit properly (not too tight or too loose) with good support and non-slip soles. I avoid high heels as much as I can now, as they shift your center of gravity and reduce stability. Similarly, completely flat shoes without arch support can cause foot fatigue and affect balance.

I keep an eye on the treads of my shoes, replacing worn shoes with smooth soles regularly. House slippers pose a particular risk, as many are loose-fitting with smooth soles that can slip off or cause tripping. I choose well-fitting slippers with non-slip soles and backs that secure them to my feet.

WEATHER AND OUTDOOR SAFETY

Weather conditions dramatically affect fall risk. Ice and snow create obvious hazards, but wet leaves, rain-slicked surfaces, and even bright sun causing glare can be dangerous. I avoid going out in icy conditions when possible; when I must venture out, I wear shoes with excellent traction, and I walk slowly. One trick I already knew is to "walk like a penguin" when it's icy out, taking small steps with my feet turned outward and keeping my body weight a little more forward than usual. One positive aspect of my osteoporosis diagnosis has been to help convince my husband that we should be snowbirds in retirement and spend winters in a tropical climate!

I'm extra cautious on escalators and moving walkways, which can be challenging even for people without balance issues. I always hold the handrail and position myself away from the sides.

When walking outdoors, I pay attention to surface changes. Curbs, uneven sidewalks, and transitions from one type of pavement to another all pose potential hazards. Poor lighting makes these hazards harder to see, so I carry a small flashlight when walking in dim conditions.

ACTIVITY MODIFICATIONS VS. COMPLETE AVOIDANCE

Learning which activities to modify versus which to avoid entirely required balancing safety with the need to maintain bone health through continued physical activity. Complete avoidance of activity often does more harm than good by accelerating bone loss and muscle weakness.

Most activities can be made safer through modifications rather than complete avoidance. I still garden, but I use raised beds to avoid bending over and choose tools with long handles to reduce bending and reaching. I don't try to weed while holding the dog's leash.

I'm also careful to hinge at the hips and not to round my spine when lifting objects from the ground; I use the muscles in my legs to help me lift.

Exercise remains crucial for my bone health, but some modifications are appropriate. Building on what I learned during my

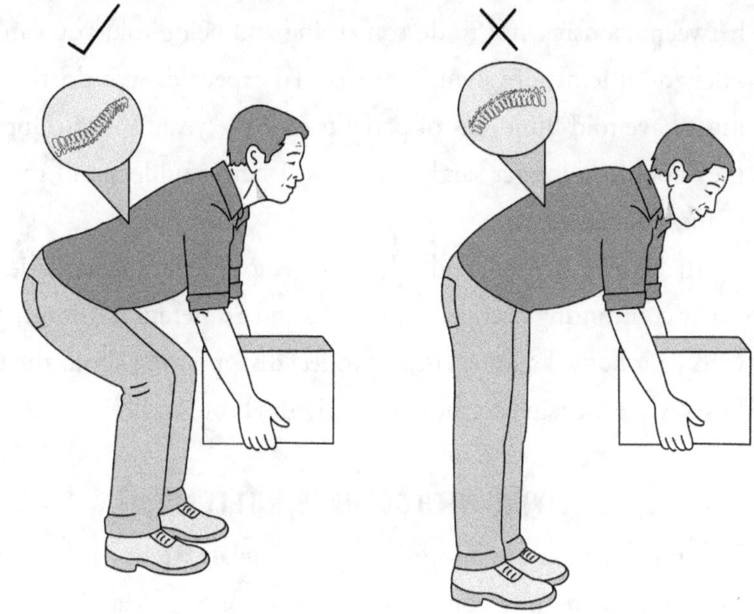

Figure 11.1: Safe lifting requires keeping the spine straight while hinging at the hips.

recovery, I avoid exercises that involve forward spine flexion with weight, or curling up of the spine during sit-ups or certain yoga movements.

THE EMOTIONAL TOLL OF RESTRICTIONS

One unexpected challenge involved grieving the loss of activities I might never do again. Even activities I rarely participated in triggered surprising sadness when I realized they were now off-limits.

I found myself mourning activities I could no longer safely do, such as roller-skating, ice-skating, skiing, and scrambling across slippery rocks with the kids in the stream (really, any spontaneous adventures involving a higher risk of falling). The difference between choosing not to do something and being told you can't safely do it felt more significant than I'd expected. As a doctor, I must have told hundreds of patients over the years about things they could no longer safely do. Now, I better understand their sadness or resistance.

This grief is normal and valid. You're not just losing activities; you're confronting changed limitations and a different relationship with your body. I allowed myself to feel disappointed about these losses while focusing on the many activities I could still enjoy safely.

LIVING WITH COURAGE, NOT FEAR

Living safely with osteoporosis requires vigilance and adaptation, but it doesn't require you to become a prisoner of fear. The goal is to maintain independence and quality of life while taking reasonable precautions to protect your bones.

I've learned to balance caution with courage, taking sensible precautions without letting osteoporosis steal more from my life than necessary. The biggest risk may not be falling; it may be becoming so afraid of falling that you stop doing the things that keep you strong, connected, and healthy.

Through trial and error, I've found ways to remain active and engaged while respecting my body's new limitations. This balance didn't come naturally; it required conscious effort and gradual rebuilding of confidence. But it's allowed me to maintain a fulfilling life while protecting my bone health and overall well-being.

The final chapter provides you with a 30-Day Action Plan designed to support you through the first month after a diagnosis.

KEY TAKEAWAYS

- The goal is balancing reasonable caution with staying active; excessive fear and inactivity worsen bone health and increase fall risk.
- Most dangerous falls happen during routine activities like nighttime bathroom trips, navigating stairs, and walking on uneven surfaces, not during dramatic activities.
- Strategic home modifications (removing throw rugs, improving lighting, installing grab bars) combined with continued physical activity provide the best protection.

CHAPTER 12

30-DAY ACTION PLAN

Finding out you have osteoporosis or osteopenia can feel overwhelming. You might be wondering where to start, what to do first, and how to prioritize the many recommendations you're receiving. This action plan will guide you through your first month, giving you concrete steps to take while you're still processing the diagnosis.

Important note: This timeline assumes you were diagnosed through screening (a DEXA scan without recent fractures). If you're reading this because you recently fractured a bone, your first priority is healing. Skip ahead to the "If You're Recovering from a Fracture" section for modified guidance that prioritizes recovery while still taking important first steps for your bone health.

WEEK 1: INFORMATION GATHERING AND ASSESSMENT

Days 1–3: Understand Your Diagnosis

Request a copy of your complete DEXA scan results, including T-scores for all tested sites (spine, hip, forearm). Ask for your Z-score as well. If available, request your FRAX or FRAXplus score. Ask about TBS if it wasn't included. Write down any questions that come up as you review your results.

Days 4–7: Schedule Essential Appointments

Make an appointment with your primary care doctor or endocrinologist to discuss treatment options (aim to do this within two to four weeks). Gather previous results if you've had relevant tests done (vitamin D level, calcium level, parathyroid hormone, thyroid function, complete blood count, kidney and liver function, bone turnover markers). If you haven't seen a dentist in the past year, schedule a dental checkup (important before starting certain bone medications).

Throughout Week 1: Start a Bone Health Journal

Record your current height (measure against a wall). List all medications and supplements you're currently taking. Note any symptoms you've been experiencing (back pain, height loss, etc.). Document your family history of osteoporosis or fractures. Track questions to ask your doctor.

WEEK 2: BEGIN SAFE LIFESTYLE CHANGES

Days 8–10: Assess Your Environment

Walk through your home looking for fall hazards (refer to Chapter 11). Make a list of safety improvements needed. Start with quick fixes: remove throw rugs, improve lighting, clear clutter from walkways. Check that you have sturdy handrails where you need them.

Days 11–14: Start Gentle Movement

If you aren't doing so already, begin walking daily, even if just for 10–15 minutes. Practice standing on one foot while holding on to a counter (work up to 30 seconds per side). Start noticing your posture throughout the day; aim to keep your tummy in and shoulders back. Avoid forward bending, twisting, or high-impact activities until you discuss exercise with your healthcare provider.

Throughout Week 2: Dietary Assessment

Track what you eat for three to four days. Calculate your approximate daily calcium intake (see Chapter 8). Note how much caffeine, alcohol, and soda you typically consume. Identify one dietary change you can make this week (example: swap afternoon soda with water, or swap potato chips with almonds).

WEEK 3: TREATMENT PLANNING AND IMPLEMENTATION

Days 15–17: Medical Appointments and Decisions

Attend your doctor's appointment with your list of questions. First, discuss whether you need screening for other medical conditions that could be causing bone loss. Review your health history and medication list for possible "hidden thieves" (see Chapter 6). Expect, at minimum, some basic blood tests, such as a metabolic panel and a Vitamin D level to be ordered. Your healthcare provider should also consider tests for: thyroid or parathyroid disease, inflammatory disease, Celiac disease, diabetes, Cushing's disease, and multiple myeloma. After testing is done and any abnormal results addressed, ask about osteoporosis treatment: Is medication recommended for your situation? Could you try diet and exercise first, and if so, when will a follow-up DEXA be done? Discuss when to start, what side effects to watch for, how long you'll need to take the medication, and the monitoring schedule.

Days 18–21: Supplement Strategy

Based on your bloodwork results, start appropriate supplements: calcium citrate (if dietary intake is insufficient), vitamin D (dosage based on your blood level), vitamin K2-MK7 (if recommended by your doctor), and magnesium (if not getting enough from diet). Consider collagen peptides (discuss with your doctor). Set up a system to remember daily supplements (phone alarm, pill organizer). Take calcium in divided doses (no more than 500 mg at once). Take calcium and vitamin D with food for better absorption.

Throughout Week 3: Medication Education

If you're prescribed medication, read all patient information carefully and consult with your pharmacist. Note the best time to take it. Understand what to do if you miss a dose. Know what side effects warrant calling your doctor. Set up reminders to take medication correctly.

WEEK 4: BUILDING YOUR SUPPORT SYSTEM AND LONG-TERM PLAN

Days 22–24: Assemble Your Healthcare Team

Identify who will manage your osteoporosis care (primary care doctor, endocrinologist, or another specialist). Ask for referrals if needed: physical therapist with osteoporosis expertise, registered dietitian, endocrinologist or rheumatologist with osteoporosis expertise. Schedule your next follow-up appointment (typically in three to six months).

Days 25–28: Exercise Program Development

If possible, schedule an appointment with a physical therapist who specializes in osteoporosis. Discuss which exercises are safe and beneficial for your specific situation. Get guidance on proper form and progression. Create a realistic weekly exercise schedule (refer to Chapter 7). Start with two to three days of strength training and daily walking per week.

Days 29–30: Create Your Ongoing Management Plan

Review what you've accomplished in the past month, and recalibrate your efforts as needed. Set three-month goals: exercise consistency target, dietary improvements, weight management goals (if applicable), fall-prevention measures completed. Mark your calendar for the following: next DEXA scan (typically in one to two years, but your doctor will advise), next medical appointment, regular medication refills, bloodwork follow-ups.

END OF MONTH: CELEBRATE YOUR PROGRESS

Take a moment to acknowledge that you've taken control of your bone health. You've moved from shock and uncertainty to active management. This is a significant accomplishment.

IF YOU'RE RECOVERING FROM A FRACTURE

Your first 30 days look different, because healing takes priority. Here's your modified plan.

Week 1: Focus on Healing and Pain Management

Follow your doctor's instructions for activity restrictions carefully. Take prescribed pain medication as directed; contact a pain management doctor if your pain is severe. Get adequate rest. Make sure you're eating enough protein and calories for healing. Start calcium and vitamin D supplementation (if not already taking). Ask about testing for other reasons for weakening of the bones. If you're younger (under 65) or have any history of cancer, it's important to ask your doctor whether more serious conditions (like cancer or multiple myeloma) could be causing your fractures.

What to skip: Don't start an exercise program yet. Don't attempt balance exercises or strength training. Avoid assessing your home for fall hazards on your own (you may not be steady enough).

Week 2: Gentle Resumption of Activity

Begin whatever gentle movement your doctor has cleared (this may be limited initially; you may be told to get moving right away or to rest as much as possible). Work with physical therapy if prescribed. Continue focusing on nutrition and healing. Start a bone health journal when you feel up to it. Don't rush recovery. Avoid any exercises that cause pain.

Week 3: Planning for Long-Term Management

Schedule or attend appointments to discuss osteoporosis treatment. Begin to address one dietary change if you're feeling better. Review medications with your doctor (some may have contributed to your fracture risk). Ask about the timeline for more active bone-strengthening exercises. Don't be surprised if you start feeling down or discouraged; find someone to talk to about your feelings.

Week 4: Building Your Foundation

If you're healing well, begin to implement home safety changes (with help). Start planning your exercise program for when you're fully healed. Focus on consistency with supplements and any prescribed medications. Set realistic expectations for your recovery timeline.

Important Reminders for Fracture Recovery

Healing varies widely by individual and fracture type. Single vertebral fractures may heal in 6–12 weeks, but multiple vertebral fractures can take much longer (sometimes a year or more). Hip fractures typically require three to six months to heal. Ask your doctor about scheduling follow-up imaging to monitor healing progress. Pain should gradually improve week by week, though the timeline varies, and you can expect pain to rebound a little bit when you start new activities. Your activity level will increase slowly under medical supervision. Some of the recommendations in this book (especially Chapter 7 on exercise) should be postponed until you're healed. Be patient with yourself; recovering from a fracture while processing an osteoporosis diagnosis is genuinely difficult.

BEYOND THE FIRST 30 DAYS

By the end of your first month, you've established the foundation. Now, the focus shifts to maintaining consistency with medications and supplements, gradually building your exercise program, making ongoing dietary improvements, attending follow-up appointments, monitoring your progress, and staying educated about updates in bone health.

Remember, managing osteoporosis is a marathon, not a sprint. The actions you take in these first 30 days set the stage for long-term bone health, but give yourself grace as you adapt to this new reality. Some days will feel overwhelming. Other days, you'll feel empowered and in control. Both responses are normal.

You're not alone on this journey, and taking action, even small steps, makes a real difference in your bone health outcomes. Keep moving forward, one day at a time.

Looking back at everything I've shared in these pages, from the shock of my diagnosis to the science of bone biology, from nutrition and exercise to medication and navigating the healthcare system, I realize that this journey has changed me in ways I never expected. I want to leave you with some final thoughts about what it truly means to be strong.

FINAL THOUGHTS

FROM FRACTURE TO STRENGTH

My journey from that unexpected fall with Finnegan to authoring this book has been one of the most challenging and transformative experiences of my life. What began as a shocking diagnosis became an opportunity to understand my body in ways I never had before, to advocate for my health more effectively, and to help others navigate the same path with knowledge and hope.

If you're reading this as someone newly diagnosed with osteoporosis or bone loss, know that you're not alone, and you're not powerless. The diagnosis may feel overwhelming initially, but it's also your opportunity to take control of your bone health in ways that can dramatically improve your future.

The science of bone health is encouraging. We have effective treatments, proven lifestyle interventions, and an understanding of bone biology that continues to advance. More importantly, we have evidence that taking action makes a real difference, not just in bone density numbers but in quality of life and confidence.

Your bones may be more fragile than you realized, but your capacity for resilience, adaptation, and strength extends far beyond your skeleton. The journey from fracture to strength isn't just about rebuilding bone; it's about rebuilding your approach to health and your vision of what's possible for your future.

Whether you're preventing your first fracture or recovering from one that's already occurred, remember that every step you take is an investment in your future self. Every calcium-rich meal, every balance exercise, every medication dose, and every safety modification isn't just about managing a condition; it's about actively creating the strongest, most resilient version of yourself possible.

Stay curious, stay engaged with your healthcare team, and, most importantly, stay hopeful. The path from diagnosis to empowerment is different for everyone, but it's a journey worth taking. Your bones, and your future self, will thank you for it.

You are strong.

FREQUENTLY ASKED QUESTIONS

GETTING STARTED AFTER DIAGNOSIS

I was just diagnosed with osteoporosis (or osteopenia). What should I do first?

Take a breath. An osteoporosis or osteopenia diagnosis can feel overwhelming, but it's manageable. Your first steps should be to get a copy of your full DEXA scan results (not just a summary), ask your doctor about your FRAX score (a fracture risk calculator). Chapter 4 walks you through how to read your DEXA results and what questions to ask, and the 30-Day Action Plan (Chapter 12) gives you a week-by-week roadmap.

What's the difference between osteopenia and osteoporosis?

Both are measured by your T-score on a DEXA scan. A T-score between –1.0 and –2.5 indicates osteopenia (mild bone loss), while –2.5 or lower indicates osteoporosis (significant bone loss). However, these are points on a spectrum, not two separate diseases. Importantly, you can still fracture with osteopenia. My own T-scores fell in the osteopenia range, yet I had four compression fractures.

That's why your fracture risk (FRAX score) matters as much as your T-score. Chapter 4 explains this in detail.

Is osteoporosis reversible? Can I rebuild bone I've already lost?

You can meaningfully improve your bone density with the right combination of exercise, nutrition, and (when appropriate) medication. Some medications, particularly anabolic drugs like teriparatide and romosozumab, actively stimulate new bone formation rather than simply slowing loss. Combined with weight-bearing exercise, resistance exercise, and proper nutrition, many people see real improvement in their DEXA scores over time. My own journey from four compression fractures back to an active life is proof that significant recovery is possible. Chapters 7, 8, and 9 cover the three pillars of rebuilding bone strength.

I feel fine. Do I really need to worry about osteoporosis?

Yes, and that's exactly what makes osteoporosis so dangerous. It's called a "silent disease" because bones weaken without any symptoms until a fracture occurs. I was active, felt healthy, and had no idea my bones were deteriorating until I fractured four vertebrae from a simple fall. Estimates suggest that one in two to one in three women over 50 will experience an osteoporotic fracture in their lifetime. Early detection through DEXA screening and proactive management are the best defenses. Chapter 1 tells my story of how an unexpected diagnosis changed everything.

Is osteoporosis hereditary? Should my children be concerned?

Family history is one of the strongest risk factors for osteoporosis.

If you've been diagnosed, your children, and especially daughters, should be aware that they may have a genetic predisposition to lower bone density. Encourage them to build the strongest possible bone bank during their younger years through weight-bearing exercise, adequate calcium and vitamin D, and avoiding bone-depleting habits. Chapter 6 covers genetic and family risk factors in depth.

UNDERSTANDING FRACTURES

I had a vertebral compression fracture, but it didn't hurt that much. Does that mean it's not serious?

Not necessarily. Many vertebral compression fractures cause little or no pain; in fact, only about one-third of vertebral fractures ever come to medical attention. Silent fractures are still serious because they weaken your spinal structure, change your posture, and substantially increase your risk of additional fractures. Research consistently shows a dose–response relationship: the more vertebrae that fracture, the higher the risks to your mobility, breathing, quality of life, and even survival. If you've been told you have an old compression fracture, even a painless one, treat it as a clear signal that your bones need attention. Chapter 5 explains the cascade effect and why that first fracture matters so much.

The mortality statistics for hip fractures are terrifying. Should I really be that scared?

I understand the fear; those numbers frightened me too when I first saw them. But context matters enormously. The often-quoted mortality figures are population averages that include very elderly, very sick people who were already at higher risk before their fracture. A relatively healthy 65-year-old woman who breaks a hip has a very different outlook from an 85-year-old man with heart disease and diabetes. Two things are true at once: fractures happen more often in sicker people, *and* fractures make people sicker. The part where fractures make people sicker (surgery complications, immobility, blood clots, deconditioning) is concentrated in the first three to six months, and that's exactly where good care and early action make the biggest difference. Chapter 5 breaks down the numbers by age and sex so you can understand your individual risk, not just the averages.

I broke my wrist in a fall. Should I be worried about osteoporosis?

Yes: a wrist fracture after a simple fall is one of the earliest warning signs of weakening bones. Wrist fractures typically occur 10–15 years before hip fractures, so they're your skeleton's early alarm system. The same is true for rib fractures and upper arm fractures near the shoulder. Don't make the mistake of thinking, "It's just a wrist." Ask your doctor to order a DEXA scan. That conversation could prevent a much more serious fracture down the road. Chapter 5 explains the different types of osteoporotic fractures and which ones serve as early warnings.

What's the "cascade effect" with osteoporotic fractures?

The cascade effect refers to how one fracture dramatically increases your risk of additional fractures. People who experience one vertebral compression fracture have a five-fold increased risk of additional spinal fractures and a two- to three-fold increased risk of hip fractures. This happens partly because structural changes from one fracture alter how forces are distributed through your skeleton, placing extra stress on other bones. It also happens because the pain, immobility, and muscle weakness that follow a fracture can accelerate bone loss and increase fall risk, creating a vicious cycle. Understanding this cascade motivated me to take my treatment seriously after my four fractures. Preventing the next fracture became just as important as recovering from the ones I already had. Chapter 5 discusses the cascade effect in detail.

Someone told me that vertebral fractures aren't as bad as hip fractures. Is that true?

People often say that to be reassuring, and I heard it too while recovering from my four compression fractures. While it's true that hip fractures carry the highest short-term mortality risk, vertebral fractures are far from minor. They increase the risk of death by about 1.5–2 times compared with similar people who haven't fractured, and they take a real toll on daily life: chronic back pain, height loss, postural changes, difficulty breathing if multiple vertebrae are involved, and significant impacts on mobility and independence. Multiple vertebral fractures compound all of these problems. Chapter 5 gives an honest look at what vertebral fractures really mean and provides five concrete steps you can take to protect your quality of life after experiencing one.

What should I do immediately after an osteoporotic fracture to give myself the best chance of recovery?

The most important steps in the first days and weeks are to get moving as soon as it's safely possible (immobility is one of the biggest threats to recovery), work with your care team on a pain management plan that keeps you functional rather than bed-bound, and start the conversation about bone-strengthening medication right away. People who begin osteoporosis treatment after a fragility fracture have fewer new fractures and significantly lower mortality than those who go untreated. Beyond those first steps, commit to rehabilitation, pay attention to your emotional health (depression and fear of falling are common and treatable), and take active steps to prevent the next fracture through fall risk reduction and maintaining your strength. Chapter 5 includes detailed "Five Ways to Protect Your Quality of Life" checklists for both vertebral and hip fractures.

UNDERSTANDING YOUR BONES AND RISK FACTORS

What causes osteoporosis? Is it just aging and menopause?

Aging and menopause are major factors, as women can lose up to 20% of their bone density in the five to seven years following menopause, but they're far from the only causes. Many everyday factors silently steal bone strength: certain medications (especially steroids), inflammatory diseases, excessive caffeine and alcohol, carbonated beverages, chronic stress, vitamin D deficiency, sedentary lifestyle, and rapid weight loss. Chapter 6 identifies over a dozen of these "hidden thieves" and explains how they work together to weaken bones.

Can men get osteoporosis?

Absolutely. While osteoporosis is more common in women, approximately one in four to one in five men over 50 will experience an osteoporotic fracture in their lifetime. Men tend to be diagnosed later because screening is less routine, which means fractures can be the first sign of a problem. The information in this book about bone biology, nutrition, exercise, and medication applies to men as well as women.

What is a DEXA scan and how do I read my results?

A DEXA (dual-energy X-ray absorptiometry) scan is a painless, low-radiation test that measures bone mineral density, usually at the hip and spine. Your results include a T-score (comparing your bones to those of a healthy 30-year-old) and a Z-score (comparing you to others your age). Chapter 4 explains exactly what these numbers mean, introduces the FRAX fracture risk calculator, and discusses additional measures like TBS that give a more complete picture of your bone health.

How often should I get a DEXA scan?

For most people with osteoporosis or osteopenia, every one to two years is typical. However, the right frequency depends on your individual situation: your current bone density, whether you're on medication, and your overall fracture risk. If you're starting a new medication, a follow-up scan at one to two years helps assess whether it's working. Chapter 4 discusses recommended screening intervals and when to push for more frequent monitoring.

EXERCISE AND OSTEOPOROSIS

What are the best exercises for osteoporosis?

The most effective exercises for building and maintaining bone density are weight-bearing exercises (walking, hiking, dancing, stair climbing) and resistance training (lifting weights, using resistance bands, bodyweight exercises). Impact and muscle-pulling forces signal your bones to grow stronger. Exercises like swimming and cycling, while great for cardiovascular health, don't load the skeleton enough to stimulate bone growth. Balance training is also essential for preventing falls. Chapter 7 provides a detailed, evidence-based exercise program with specific recommendations for beginners through advanced exercisers.

Are there exercises I should avoid with osteoporosis?

Generally, you should avoid high-impact activities that involve sudden jarring (like jumping on hard surfaces), heavy forward bending or rounding of the spine under load, and twisting movements with force, especially if you have vertebral fractures. However, the goal is modification, not total avoidance. Many activities can be adapted to be safe. Working with a physical therapist who specializes in osteoporosis is ideal, but Chapter 7 also provides guidance for those who don't have access to a specialist.

I'm afraid of falling and breaking a bone. How do I stay active without being reckless?

This fear is incredibly common and completely understandable. Ironically, becoming less active out of fear actually weakens your bones and muscles further, increasing your fall risk. The key is building strength and balance progressively while taking smart precautions. Chapter 11 covers fall-prevention strategies for your home and daily life, and Chapter 7 includes balance exercises that reduce fall risk. The goal is living with courage, not fear.

NUTRITION AND BONE HEALTH

What are the best food sources of calcium for bone health?

Dairy products remain excellent sources: one cup of Greek yogurt provides about 250 mg of calcium, and a glass of milk about 300 mg. For non-dairy options, sardines with bones (380 mg per small can), calcium-fortified plant milks (check labels, as amounts vary dramatically between brands), tofu made with calcium sulfate, almonds, broccoli, kale, and bok choy are all good choices. The goal for most adults is 1,000–1,200 mg of calcium daily from food and supplements combined.[84] Chapter 8 includes a comprehensive "Strong Bones Food List" organized by food category, with calcium content for each item.

Should I take calcium supplements? What kind is best?

Food sources are always preferable, but supplements can fill the gap if your diet falls short. Calcium citrate is generally recommended, because it can be taken with or without food and is better absorbed, especially if you're taking acid-reducing medications. Calcium carbonate is less expensive but must be taken with food for proper absorption. Avoid taking more than 500 mg of supplemental calcium at one time, as your body cannot absorb more than that in a single dose. Chapter 8 discusses supplement timing, dosing, and what to look for.

How much vitamin D do I need, and how do I know if I'm deficient?

Most osteoporosis experts recommend maintaining a blood level of 40–50 ng/mL of vitamin D. Many people need 2,000–5,000 IU daily to reach and maintain this level, though the right dose depends on your current blood level, body weight, and sun exposure. The only way to know your level is through a simple blood test (25-hydroxyvitamin D). Vitamin D is essential because, without it, your body cannot properly absorb calcium. Chapter 8 covers the complete vitamin D equation, including food sources, supplementation, and monitoring.

Are there foods that are bad for my bones?

Yes. Excessive caffeine, alcohol, and sodium all increase calcium loss. Ultra-processed foods containing phosphate additives can interfere with calcium absorption. Carbonated beverages, particularly colas, have been associated with lower bone density. This doesn't mean you must eliminate these foods entirely, but awareness and moderation matter. Chapter 6 covers dietary "bone thieves" in detail, and Chapter 8 offers practical substitutions that are both bone-friendly and enjoyable.

MEDICATION QUESTIONS

Do I really need medication for osteoporosis, or can I manage it with diet and exercise alone?

It depends on your fracture risk. If you've already fractured, or if your FRAX score indicates high risk, lifestyle changes alone are usually not enough. Medication can reduce fracture risk by 40–70% depending on the type. Think of it this way: exercise and nutrition build the foundation, but medication provides powerful reinforcement when your bone bank is seriously depleted. Chapter 9 helps you understand when medication is recommended and how to weigh the benefits against the risks.

What are the main types of osteoporosis medications, and how do they work?

There are three main categories. Antiresorptive medications (bisphosphonates like alendronate, risedronate, and zoledronic acid, plus denosumab) slow bone breakdown by calming the cells that remove old bone. Anabolic medications (teriparatide, abaloparatide, and romosozumab) stimulate new bone formation by activating bone-building cells. Hormonal therapies (raloxifene and estrogen) work through hormone-related pathways to protect bone. Chapter 9 explains each type in detail, including how they're taken, common side effects, and what to expect.

I've heard bisphosphonates can cause jaw problems. Should I be worried?

Osteonecrosis of the jaw is a real but very rare side effect of bisphosphonates, occurring in roughly 1 in 100,000 to 1 in 1,000 patients taking oral bisphosphonates, with risk increasing with longer duration of use. The risk is significantly higher with intravenous bisphosphonates, which are used for cancer treatment at much higher doses than those used for osteoporosis. Good dental hygiene and completing major dental work before starting treatment can further reduce this already small risk. Chapter 9 puts this and other medication risks in perspective, helping you make an informed decision rather than one based on fear.

What's a "drug holiday," and will I need one?

After three to five years on bisphosphonates (or longer, depending on your risk level), your doctor may suggest a temporary pause called a "drug holiday." This is because bisphosphonates accumulate in bone and continue working for some time after you stop taking them. During a drug holiday, your bone density is monitored; afterward, treatment resumes if needed. Not all medications allow for drug holidays. Denosumab, for example, should never be stopped abruptly without transitioning to another medication, as rapid bone loss can follow. Chapter 9 discusses treatment duration, drug holidays, and sequential treatment strategies.

How long does it take for osteoporosis medication to work?

Most medications begin working at the cellular level within weeks, but measurable changes on a DEXA scan typically take one to two years to appear. Fracture risk reduction begins before density changes are visible on scans. This means the medication is protecting you even before your numbers improve. Chapter 9 covers realistic treatment timelines and what to expect during the first months and years of therapy.

WORKING WITH YOUR HEALTHCARE TEAM

What type of doctor should I see for osteoporosis?

Several types of specialists treat osteoporosis: endocrinologists, rheumatologists, orthopedic specialists, and physiatrists (physical medicine and rehabilitation doctors). A physiatrist actually made my diagnosis. Some gynecologists and internists also have expertise in bone health. The most important thing is finding a provider who takes osteoporosis seriously, orders comprehensive testing, and stays current on treatment options. Chapter 10 covers how to find the right specialist and what red flags to watch for in your care.

My doctor says my osteopenia is "nothing to worry about." Should I get a second opinion?

If you have risk factors for fracture (family history, previous fracture, early menopause, long-term steroid use, or other factors), dismissing osteopenia may not be appropriate. A FRAX score can help clarify your actual fracture risk beyond just your T-score. If your concerns are being brushed aside, seeking a second opinion from a bone health specialist is absolutely reasonable. Chapter 10 discusses when and how to advocate for yourself and when to seek another perspective.

LIVING WITH OSTEOPOROSIS

How do I make my home safer to prevent falls?

Start with the highest-risk areas: remove loose rugs or secure them with non-slip backing, improve lighting (especially in hallways, stairs, and bathrooms), install grab bars in the shower and near the toilet, keep floors clear of clutter and cords, and make sure stair railings are sturdy. Wear supportive shoes with non-slip soles, even indoors.

How do I cope with the emotional impact of an osteoporosis diagnosis?

The emotional toll is real and often underestimated. Fear, grief, frustration, and anxiety are all normal responses. I experienced every one of them. What helped me most was acknowledging these feelings rather than pushing them aside, educating myself to replace fear with knowledge, connecting with others who understood, and gradually rebuilding confidence through small physical victories. Chapter 2 is devoted entirely to the emotional journey, from the initial shock through building resilience, because emotional health is just as important as physical treatment.

I have osteoporosis. Can I still travel, work, play with my children or grandchildren, and live a full life?

Yes. Osteoporosis requires adjustments, not a life sentence of restriction. With proper treatment, smart precautions, and continued strength and balance training, most people with osteoporosis can remain active and engaged. I went from four compression fractures and months in a back brace to hiking, traveling, and living fully again. The key is learning which activities to modify and which precautions to take, rather than retreating from life. Chapter 11 covers activity modifications, and the entire book is built around the idea that you can be strong in spirit, even when your bones need extra care.

GLOSSARY OF MEDICAL TERMS

The medical terminology in this book can be challenging to pronounce. This glossary provides pronunciation guides and brief definitions for key terms used throughout the book.

Abaloparatide (a-bal-oh-PAR-ah-tide): An anabolic (bone-building) medication (brand name Tymlos) given as a daily injection.

Alendronate (ah-LEN-droe-nate): A bisphosphonate medication (brand name Fosamax) taken orally to treat osteoporosis.

Bisphosphonates (bis-FOS-foe-nates): A class of medications that slow bone loss by inhibiting osteoclast activity.

Cancellous bone (KAN-sell-us): The spongy, honeycomb-like interior bone tissue; also called trabecular bone.

Calcitonin (kal-sih-TOE-nin): A naturally occurring hormone that slows bone breakdown. Synthetic salmon calcitonin was once prescribed as a nasal spray for osteoporosis, but it has largely been replaced by more effective medications.

Denosumab (den-OH-sue-mab): A biologic medication (brand name Prolia) given by injection every six months to slow bone loss.

Estrogen (ES-troh-jen): A hormone that plays a key role in maintaining bone density. Estrogen therapy, sometimes combined with other agents, is used to prevent bone loss in postmenopausal women.

Hyperparathyroidism (high-per-para-THY-royd-ism): A condition in which one or more parathyroid glands produce too much parathyroid hormone, leading to increased bone breakdown.

Ibandronate (eye-BAN-droe-nate): A *bisphosphonate* medication (brand name Boniva) available in monthly oral or quarterly intravenous forms.

Kyphoplasty (KYE-foe-plas-tee): A minimally invasive procedure to treat vertebral compression fractures by inflating a balloon in the fractured vertebra and filling it with bone cement.

Kyphosis (kye-FOE-sis): An exaggerated forward curvature of the upper spine, sometimes called a "dowager's hump."

Osteoblasts (OS-tee-oh-blasts): Bone-building cells that create new bone tissue.

Osteoclasts (OS-tee-oh-clasts): Bone-resorbing cells that break down old or damaged bone tissue.

Osteopenia (os-tee-oh-PEE-nee-ah): A condition of mildly reduced bone density, between normal bone density and osteoporosis.

Osteoporosis (os-tee-oh-pore-OH-sis): A condition in which bones become weak and brittle due to loss of bone density and mass.

Physiatrist (fiz-EYE-ah-trist): A physician specializing in physical medicine and rehabilitation, trained to diagnose and treat conditions affecting the muscles, bones, nerves, and brain without surgery.

Raloxifene (ral-OX-ih-feen): A selective estrogen receptor modulator (SERM) used to prevent and treat osteoporosis in postmenopausal women.

Risedronate (rih-SEH-droe-nate): A *bisphosphonate* medication (brand name Actonel) taken orally to treat osteoporosis.

Romosozumab (roe-moe-SOE-zoo-mab): A dual-action medication (brand name Evenity) given as a monthly injection that both builds new bone and slows bone loss.

Teriparatide (ter-ih-PAR-ah-tide): An anabolic (bone-building) medication (brand name Forteo) given as a daily injection.

Thoracic (thor-AS-ik): Relating to the chest region of the spine (the 12 vertebrae between the neck and lower back).

Trabecular bone (trah-BEK-you-lar): See *cancellous bone*.

Vertebrae (VER-teh-bray): The individual bones that make up the spinal column.

Vertebroplasty (ver-TEE-bro-plas-tee): A minimally invasive procedure to treat vertebral compression fractures by injecting bone cement directly into the fractured vertebra to stabilize it. Unlike *kyphoplasty*, no balloon is used to restore height before the cement is injected.

Zoledronic acid (zoe-leh-DRON-ik): A bisphosphonate medication (brand name Reclast) given as an annual intravenous infusion.

NOTES

1. International Osteoporosis Foundation. "Epidemiology of osteoporosis and fragility fractures." https://www.osteoporosis.foundation/facts-statistics/epidemiology-of-osteoporosis-and-fragility-fractures
2. International Osteoporosis Foundation, "Epidemiology of osteoporosis."
3. Bone Health and Osteoporosis Foundation. "What women need to know." https://www.bonehealthandosteoporosis.org/preventing-fractures/general-facts/what-women-need-to-know/
4. Bone Health and Osteoporosis Foundation. "Just for men." https://www.bonehealthandosteoporosis.org/preventing-fractures/general-facts/just-for-men/
5. Kiebzak GM, et al. "Underdiagnosis of osteoporosis in men." Endocrine Practice, 2002. https://pmc.ncbi.nlm.nih.gov/articles/PMC7755710/
6. Sheehan KJ, et al. "Patient and system factors of mortality after hip fracture: a scoping review." BMC Geriatrics, 2016. https://pubmed.ncbi.nlm.nih.gov/27079195/
7. Choksi P, et al. "The challenges of diagnosing osteoporosis and the limitations of currently available tools." Endocrine Practice, 2018. https://pmc.ncbi.nlm.nih.gov/articles/PMC7755710/
8. Manolagas SC, Parfitt AM. "What old means to bone." Trends in Endocrinology & Metabolism, 2010. https://pmc.ncbi.nlm.nih.gov/articles/PMC2880220/
9. Kenkre JS, Bassett JHD. "The bone remodelling cycle." Annals of Clinical Biochemistry, 2018. https://pubmed.ncbi.nlm.nih.gov/29368538/
10. Kenkre and Bassett, "The bone remodelling cycle."
11. Weaver CM, et al. "The National Osteoporosis Foundation's position statement on peak bone mass development and lifestyle factors.". Osteoporosis International, 2016. https://pubmed.ncbi.nlm.nih.gov/26856587/
12. Baxter-Jones AD, et al. "Bone mineral accrual from 8 to 30 years of age." Sports Health, 2020. https://pmc.ncbi.nlm.nih.gov/articles/PMC7485021/
13. Bone Health and Osteoporosis Foundation, "What women need to know."

14. Looker AC, et al. "Updated data on proximal femur bone mineral levels of US adults." Osteoporosis International, 1998. https://pubmed.ncbi.nlm.nih.gov/12049882/

15. International Osteoporosis Foundation, "Epidemiology of osteoporosis."

16. Dyer SM, et al. "A critical review of the long-term disability outcomes following hip fracture." BMC Geriatrics, 2016. https://pmc.ncbi.nlm.nih.gov/articles/PMC5010762/

17. Sarafrazi N, et al. "Osteoporosis or low bone mass in older adults: United States, 2017–2018." CDC NCHS Data Brief No. 405, 2021. https://www.cdc.gov/nchs/products/databriefs/db405.htm

18. Wright NC, et al. "The recent prevalence of osteoporosis and low bone mass." JBMR, 2014. https://pmc.ncbi.nlm.nih.gov/articles/PMC4757905/

19. Pasco JA, et al. "The population burden of fractures originates in women with osteopenia." Osteoporosis International, 2006. https://pubmed.ncbi.nlm.nih.gov/16699736/

20. Kreiger N, et al. "The Canadian Multicentre Osteoporosis Study (CaMos)." Canadian Journal on Aging, 1999. https://pubmed.ncbi.nlm.nih.gov/11199195/

21. FRAX® Fracture Risk Assessment Tool. University of Sheffield. https://frax.shef.ac.uk/

22. "Vertebral Compression Fractures." StatPearls, National Library of Medicine. https://www.ncbi.nlm.nih.gov/books/NBK448171/

23. Center JR, et al. "Mortality after all major types of osteoporotic fracture in men and women." Lancet, 1999. https://pubmed.ncbi.nlm.nih.gov/10093978/

24. Bliuc D, et al. "Mortality risk associated with low-trauma osteoporotic fracture." JAMA, 2009. https://pubmed.ncbi.nlm.nih.gov/19594305/

25. Lyles KW, et al. "Zoledronic acid and clinical fractures and mortality after hip fracture." NEJM, 2007. https://pubmed.ncbi.nlm.nih.gov/17989383/

26. CDC HCUP Data. "Hip fracture hospitalizations, 2019." https://stacks.cdc.gov/view/cdc/126881

27. Sheehan et al., "Patient and system factors of mortality after hip fracture."

28. Guzon-Illescas O, et al. "Mortality after osteoporotic hip fracture: incidence, trends, and associated factors." Journal of Orthopaedic Surgery and Research, 2019. https://pubmed.ncbi.nlm.nih.gov/31272470/

29. Dyer et al., "Long-term disability outcomes following hip fracture."

30. Zhao JG, et al. "The efficacy of bisphosphonates for prevention of osteoporotic fracture." Journal of Bone Metabolism, 2017. https://pmc.ncbi.nlm.nih.gov/articles/PMC5357611/

31. International Osteoporosis Foundation: Bisphosphonates Treatment Page. https://www.osteoporosis.foundation/health-professionals/treatment/bisphosphonates

32. Court-Brown CM, Caesar B. "Epidemiology of adult fractures." Journal of Bone and Joint Surgery, 2006. https://pubmed.ncbi.nlm.nih.gov/17142295/

33. Lindsay R, et al. "Risk of new vertebral fracture in the year following a fracture." JAMA, 2001. https://pubmed.ncbi.nlm.nih.gov/11176842/

34. Weinstein RS. "Glucocorticoid-induced osteoporosis and osteonecrosis." Endocrinology and Metabolism Clinics, 2012. https://pmc.ncbi.nlm.nih.gov/articles/PMC3417039/

35. Devogelaer JP, et al. "Glucocorticoid-induced osteoporosis: a review." Clinical and Experimental Rheumatology, 2006. https://pubmed.ncbi.nlm.nih.gov/16217586/

36. Weinstein, "Glucocorticoid-induced osteoporosis and osteonecrosis."

37. Devogelaer et al., "Glucocorticoid-induced osteoporosis: a review."

38. Brody DJ, Gu Q. "Antidepressant use among adults: United States, 2015–2018." CDC NCHS Data Brief No. 377, 2020. https://www.cdc.gov/nchs/data/databriefs/db377-h.pdf

39. Hu J, et al. "Osteoporosis and fracture risk associated with novel antidepressants: a systematic review and meta-analysis." Ann Epidemiol Prev, 2024. https://pubmed.ncbi.nlm.nih.gov/38863057/

40. de Filippis R, et al. "Antidepressants and vertebral and hip risk fracture: an updated systematic review and meta-analysis." Healthcare, 2022. https://pubmed.ncbi.nlm.nih.gov/35627940/

41. Alsugeir D, et al. "Risk of osteoporotic fractures in menopausal women with common mental health diagnoses prescribed SSRIs/SNRIs: cohort and self-controlled case series analyses." Arch Osteoporosis, 2024. https://doi.org/10.1007/s11657-024-01459-3

42. Silverberg SJ, Bilezikian JP. "Primary hyperparathyroidism." The Permanente Journal, 2001. https://pmc.ncbi.nlm.nih.gov/articles/PMC3042336/

43. Giordano R, Parasiliti Caprino M, Loli P, Giustina A. "Screening for endogenous hypercortisolism in patients with osteoporosis and fracture." Journal of Endocrinological Investigation. 2024;48(Suppl 1):23-31.

44. Wippert PM, Rector M, Kuhn G, Wuertz-Kozak K. "Stress and Alterations in Bones: An Interdisciplinary Perspective." Frontiers in Endocrinology. 2017;8:96.

45. Schwartz AV, Vittinghoff E, Bauer DC, et al. "Association of BMD and FRAX Score With Risk of Fracture in Older Adults With Type 2 Diabetes." JAMA. 2011;305(21):2184–2192.

46. Leslie WD, Rubin MR, Schwartz AV, Kanis JA. "Type 2 diabetes and bone." Journal of Bone and Mineral Research. 2012;27(2):301–308.

47. Centers for Disease Control and Prevention. "Chronic Kidney Disease in the United States, 2026." Atlanta, GA: US Department of Health and Human Services, Centers for Disease Control and Prevention; 2026.

48. Forrest KY, Stuhldreher WL. "Prevalence and correlates of vitamin D deficiency." Nutrition Research, 2011. https://pubmed.ncbi.nlm.nih.gov/21310306/

49. Watson SL, et al. "High-Intensity Resistance and Impact Training (LIFTMOR)." JBMR, 2018. https://pubmed.ncbi.nlm.nih.gov/28975661/

50. Umemura Y, et al. "Five jumps per day increase bone mass and breaking force in rats." JBMR, 1997. https://pubmed.ncbi.nlm.nih.gov/12235034/

51. Umemura et al., "Five jumps per day increase bone mass and breaking force in rats."

52. Sherrington C, et al. "Exercise for preventing falls in older people." Cochrane Database, 2019. https://pubmed.ncbi.nlm.nih.gov/30703272/

53. Zhao R, et al. "Effectiveness of exercise interventions on balance and fall prevention." Frontiers in Public Health, 2023. https://pmc.ncbi.nlm.nih.gov/articles/PMC10435089/

54. Institute of Medicine. "Dietary reference intakes for calcium and vitamin D." National Academies Press, 2011. https://nap.nationalacademies.org/catalog/13050/dietary-reference-intakes-for-calcium-and-vitamin-d

55. König D, et al. "Specific collagen peptides improve bone mineral density." Nutrients, 2018. https://pubmed.ncbi.nlm.nih.gov/29337906/

56. Tripkovic L, et al. "Comparison of vitamin D2 and vitamin D3 supplementation." AJCN, 2012. https://pmc.ncbi.nlm.nih.gov/articles/PMC3349454/

57. Tangpricha V, Holick MF. "Calcium and vitamin D: Skeletal and extraskeletal health." Current Rheumatology Reports, 2008. https://pmc.ncbi.nlm.nih.gov/articles/PMC2669834/

58. Institute of Medicine, "Dietary reference intakes for calcium and vitamin D."

59. Heaney RP, Weaver CM. "Calcium absorption from kale." American Journal of Clinical Nutrition, 1990. https://pubmed.ncbi.nlm.nih.gov/2321572/

60. Weaver CM, Proulx WR, Heaney R. "Choices for achieving adequate dietary calcium with a vegetarian diet." AJCN, 1999. https://pubmed.ncbi.nlm.nih.gov/10479229/

61. De Souza MJ, et al. "Prunes preserve hip bone mineral density." AJCN, 2022. https://pubmed.ncbi.nlm.nih.gov/35798020/

62. Zhao et al., "Efficacy of bisphosphonates for prevention of osteoporotic fracture."

63. International Osteoporosis Foundation, Bisphosphonates Treatment Page.

64. Black DM, et al. "Atypical femur fracture risk versus fragility fracture prevention with bisphosphonates." N Engl J Med, 2020. https://pubmed.ncbi.nlm.nih.gov/32813950/

65. Zhao et al., "Efficacy of bisphosphonates for prevention of osteoporotic fracture."

66. AAOMS. "Medication-related osteonecrosis of the jaw—2022 update." https://aaoms.org/wp-content/uploads/2024/03/mronj_position_paper.pdf

67. Khan AA, et al. "Bisphosphonate associated osteonecrosis of the jaw." Canadian Family Physician, 2008. https://pmc.ncbi.nlm.nih.gov/articles/PMC2464788/

68. Dodson TB. "The frequency of medication-related osteonecrosis of the jaw." Oral and Maxillofacial Surgery Clinics, 2015. https://pmc.ncbi.nlm.nih.gov/articles/PMC5565873/

69. Lo JC, et al. "Prevalence of osteonecrosis of the jaw in patients with oral bisphosphonate exposure." Journal of Oral and Maxillofacial Surgery, 2010. https://pmc.ncbi.nlm.nih.gov/articles/PMC10159647/

70. "Teriparatide." StatPearls, National Library of Medicine. https://www.ncbi.nlm.nih.gov/books/NBK559248/

71. Miller PD, et al. "Effect of abaloparatide on new vertebral fractures" (ACTIVE trial). JAMA, 2016. https://pubmed.ncbi.nlm.nih.gov/27533157/

72. Saag KG, et al. "Romosozumab or alendronate for fracture prevention in women with osteoporosis." NEJM, 2017. https://pubmed.ncbi.nlm.nih.gov/28892457/

73. Cosman F, et al. "Romosozumab treatment in postmenopausal women with osteoporosis" (FRAME trial). NEJM, 2016. https://www.nejm.org/doi/full/10.1056/NEJMoa1607948

74. Ettinger B, et al. "Reduction of vertebral fracture risk with raloxifene" (MORE trial). JAMA, 1999. https://pubmed.ncbi.nlm.nih.gov/10442472/

75. Ettinger et al., "Reduction of vertebral fracture risk with raloxifene."

76. Ettinger et al., "Reduction of vertebral fracture risk with raloxifene."

77. WHI Investigators. "Risks and benefits of estrogen plus progestin." JAMA, 2002. https://pubmed.ncbi.nlm.nih.gov/12117397/

78. WHI Investigators, "Risks and benefits of estrogen plus progestin."

79. WHI Investigators, "Risks and benefits of estrogen plus progestin."

80. Overman RA, et al. "Salmon calcitonin use and associated cancer risk." Ann Pharmacother, 2013. https://pubmed.ncbi.nlm.nih.gov/24259626/

81. Nakayama A, et al. "Evidence of effectiveness of a fracture liaison service." Osteoporosis International, 2016. https://pmc.ncbi.nlm.nih.gov/articles/PMC4767862/

82. Scheffer AC, et al. "Fear of falling: measurement strategy, prevalence." Age and Ageing, 2008. https://pubmed.ncbi.nlm.nih.gov/18349012/

83. Schoene D, et al. "A systematic review on the influence of fear of falling on quality of life." Clinical Interventions in Aging, 2019. https://pmc.ncbi.nlm.nih.gov/articles/PMC6514257/

84. NIH Office of Dietary Supplements: Calcium Fact Sheet for Health Professionals. https://ods.od.nih.gov/factsheets/Calcium-HealthProfessional/

ABOUT THE AUTHOR

Dr. Lisa Pocius is a board-certified family medicine physician with over 20 years of experience caring for patients. She currently serves as the medical director for a large company. When she was diagnosed with osteoporosis and multiple vertebral fractures herself, she did what any determined doctor would do: she dove headfirst into the research and asked every question she could think of. Then she decided to write the book she wished someone had handed her on diagnosis day.

Lisa lives in the Midwest with her loving family and a menagerie of beloved pets, including Finnegan, the goofy goldendoodle whose leash-pulling antics set this whole story in motion. She believes that a good attitude and a genuine love for life are every bit as important as good medicine.

For additional resources and articles on bone health, visit Dr. Pocius's website at **www.mybone.health**

www.ingramcontent.com/pod-product-compliance
Lightning Source LLC
LaVergne TN
LVHW022207200926
848481LV00006B/1880